Stress Management

Simple Techniques to Kill Your Anxiety and Be Happy

(Reduce Your Depression While Seeing Your Life in a New Light)

James Crawford

Published By **John Kembrey**

James Crawford

All Rights Reserved

Stress Management: Simple Techniques to Kill Your Anxiety and Be Happy (Reduce Your Depression While Seeing Your Life in a New Light)

ISBN 978-1-77485-548-5

No part of this guidebook shall be reproduced in any form without permission in writing from the publisher except in the case of brief quotations embodied in critical articles or reviews.

Legal & Disclaimer

The information contained in this ebook is not designed to replace or take the place of any form of medicine or professional medical advice. The information in this ebook has been provided for educational & entertainment purposes only.

The information contained in this book has been compiled from sources deemed reliable, and it is accurate to the best of the Author's knowledge; however, the Author cannot guarantee its accuracy and validity and cannot be held liable for any errors or omissions. Changes are periodically made to this book. You must consult your doctor or get professional medical advice before using any of the suggested remedies, techniques, or information in this book.

Upon using the information contained in this book, you agree to hold harmless the Author from and against any damages, costs, and expenses, including any legal fees potentially resulting from the application of any of the information provided by this guide. This disclaimer applies to any damages or injury caused by the use and application, whether directly or indirectly, of any advice or information presented, whether for breach of contract, tort, negligence, personal injury, criminal intent, or under any other cause of action.

You agree to accept all risks of using the information presented inside this book. You need to consult a professional medical practitioner in order to ensure you are both able and healthy enough to participate in this program.

TABLE OF CONTENTS

Chapter 1: What Is Stress? 1

Chapter 2: Taking Control By Letting Go .. 8

Chapter 3: Limiting Beliefs Are The Most Often Cited Cause Of Stress 12

Chapter 4: Watching What You Eat 27

Chapter 5: Strategies To Manage Your Thoughts To Control Anxiety 31

Chapter 6: Your Lifetime Relaxation Techniques 49

Chapter 7: Thinking Restructurally To Reduce Stress 54

Chapter 8: Sleeping Well-Being 59

Chapter 9: Learning Positive Attitude Tips To Declutter Your Mind 71

Chapter 10: Relaxation Techniques 88

Chapter 11: Make Care Of Yourself And Be Happy Every Minute Of Your Life 99

Chapter 12: Control And Management Of Stress 105

Chapter 13: De-Stress Your Body, Mind And Soul.. 112

Chapter 14: Redirecting Stress To Good 120

Chapter 15: Strategies To Effectively Deal With Changes And Obstacles In Life And At Work.. 138

Chapter 16: Control Your Environment Control Of Your Environment............... 147

Chapter 17: De-Stress Your Soul And Mind Control Your Thoughts 150

Chapter 18: Continue Activities With Positive 165

Chapter 19: Reaching Out 173

Conclusion 184

Chapter 1: What Is Stress?

Stress is a problem that everyone is confronted with at one point or some other time. In reality, stress is something that is a constant throughout our lives, frequently, sometimes with no knowledge. Stress in its worst form can completely turn our lives around, resulting in serious problems like anxiety breakdowns and deadly heart attacks. It is therefore crucial to understand how to spot the signs of stress, to identify triggers for stress and then find ways to control these triggers to live a happy, fulfilled life and happy.

What exactly is stress? Stress is the normal response of your body in response to any type of expectation or need. Bad and good experiences as well as demands on your mind and body could result in stress. When someone is under stress there are certain chemicals released through the body's bloodstream. These hormones - or chemicals as they are called can help an individual manage the stress circumstance by increasing their physical and mental strength. This is beneficial in times of physical danger, such as the threat of attack from an animal that is wild, etc.

But, if the stress situations are triggered by thoughts and emotions this could be harmful. The additional strength produced by the body in these kinds of stressful situations does not have an outlet in the outside world and may accumulate within the system. Stress from physical risk could be harmful in the event that it continues for a long period of time.

The causes of stress

Survival Stress - If you're afraid of injury physically the survival stress is brought into the picture. The reaction to this type or stress can be the most frequent thing that happens to living creatures that is, your body will automatically go into fight or flight mode to survive. The release of energy in this period can be extremely beneficial.

Internal Stress : This type of stress is of course is the result of anxiety that has no reason. Internal stress is a condition that people put on themselves. It's caused by anxiety about issues that are out of their control. Controlling stress within is perhaps the most challenging aspect of managing stress.

Environmental Stress is caused by through the environment you live in , such as pollution, noise crowding, etc.

Overwork-related fatigue The fatigue can build up over time, and can take an enormous burden in your physical and mental health. This type of stress is caused by overworking at work and/or at home.

What are the reasons we should control stress? What suggestions and tips can you expect from this book about stress management? Check it out to find out.

Stress can be described as the body's response to demands or pressures in life It is triggered by the result of a bad or good experience. The way it works is that when an event or change happens to you and you be stressed, and your body responds by releasing chemicals into the bloodstream. These chemicals are intended to boost your energy and strength which is a great idea if you're experiencing stress caused by physical danger, but it can be dangerous when stress is a reaction to a stressful situation. This is because when you're when there is physical danger, additional energy and strength may be released, however when you are feeling emotional, you don't be able to release it. This is why you'll notice that the accumulation of chemical and energy can result in chronic stress.

It is important to know that regardless of stress of any kind the body will have an auto-response. The body's response is usually controlled by a component that is part of our nervous system that is referred by the name of autonomic nerve system. The system is divided into two groups: the parasympathetic and sympathetic. The sympathetic regulates the response to stress, while the parasympathetic regulates the relaxing response. When there is a alteration or demand your sympathetic nerve system communicates to various areas of the body, including organs, glands, and muscles. Through this process, our bodies respond and chemical substances such as cortisol, aldosterone and adrenaline are released.

The body's chemical makeup is affected in a variety of ways, such as the increase in blood pressure, heart rate as well as stomach acid accumulation blood vessel spasms and muscle tension, among other symptoms. While these changes are adaptable and help be prepared for dealing with stress, they could lead to illness when stress becomes chronic. This is the reason why it is imperative to focus in the need for managing stress as if it is left unchecked, it could cause chronic health issues. The sooner one can relieve stress, the more healthy and happy they are and also lowers the chance of developing heart issues. The concept behind stress management is to allow the parasympathetic nervous system eliminate the effects of stress and induce relaxation and recovery throughout the body.

A majority of stress stems from worries, fears and regrets, negative thoughts as well as self-criticism and expectations. It is crucial to realize that the level of stress a person experiences is usually determined by how you view the stressor rather than by the actual stressor. That is a return to the question of how you respond to circumstances or events regardless of how challenging they may appear. All of the challenges and obstacles are part of the daily routine however, the more that you attach your feelings and emotions to them, the worse you will end up feeling.

Buddhism is a great way to learn. It states that there is no permanent thing in this world and that all your problems or struggles will pass. Therefore, it is your responsibility to ensure that your thoughts aren't affected by forces outside of your control. Let go of any negativity and that includes changing negative thoughts into positive ones. Anyone who is devoted to their life sufficiently is aware that happiness is always the top priority. It's all about making the effort necessary to be able to attain it even in the darkest of moments. Do not let stress take over your life because it can not only make you sad but can also impact your overall well-being.

Everyone needs to be aware that stress is an issue that affects every person at one moment throughout their life. Understanding when you're experiencing stress, what is the cause and various methods of dealing with stress will greatly improve your mental, emotional and physical wellbeing. The entire spectrum of information is covered in the lessons on stress management that cover an array of strategies focused on reducing stress levels. This is especially true in the case of constant stress. If you can manage stress effectively you'll have taken the first step toward improving your the quality of your life. Being in your comfort zone isn't negative, since it makes you be more effective under pressure, and it also encourages you to be more productive. If it becomes too much and stops you from functioning at a regular pace, then it's an issue. This is because it deprives you of your joy, and affects your relationships, and can affect your productivity. It is therefore important to know that managing stress efficiently, managing it effectively and understanding how to manage unhealthy stress are crucial life skills we all require. It is true that stress tension, anxiety, and stress are all commonplace in life isn't a reason to ignore these issues or believe that they'll disappear by themselves. You must be proactive by seeking aid and speaking to those who can assist you.

I hope that now you know what stress is really about, and are prepared to learn more about its prevention and treatment.

Chapter 2: Taking Control By Letting Go

Now is the time to shift our focus to the stresses that we don't have control. Have you ever made your list of stressful events that were that are beyond your control earlier? I'd like you to look at the list, and acknowledge that those problems are not in your control, and that's okay. It's fine to not have complete control over all aspects in your daily life. It's fine for you to have no solution to solve every issue. Humans are human, and it's okay to be human too. Recognizing that stresses are not your own is part of regaining control over the level of stress you experience and your mental well-being and ultimately, your entire life.

I realize that the notion of taking back control of your life through voluntarily letting go of your efforts to manage an array of stressors that cause you anxiety may seem like an absurd notion. When you take a conscious choice to release the tensions, worries or fears caused by the stressors that are uncontrollable You are also making the conscious choice to control the way your stressors impact your life. It is, in essence it's a way of regaining your authority over your own psyche, a psyche that is constantly stricken by constant concerns, worries and thoughts about stressors that are not managed. Our minds are conditioned to be constantly tackling problems which is why recognizing things as outside our realm of influence and then letting go of it may not occur easily. Here are some ideas to help you let go of your grip on these overwhelming tensions.

Relax and unwind.

We're usually caught to our anxieties about the things that stress us that we are unable to realize how to unwind. Relaxation is a distant idea, only for those who have more time and less things to do. Yet, learning how to relax is crucial for letting off the habit that is constantly pondering ways to handle stressors that you are unable to alter. Healthguide.org is a site that is dedicated to helping people who have health issues, and they have put together a complete list of relaxation methods to help relieve stress.

Learn to be flexible

The list of the stressors you're not able to manage isn't going to get any shorter as your life gets more complicated. Stress is aspect of everyday life and, as such it is imperative to incorporate the ability to adapt as part of our strategy to minimize the impact that stress has on us. Adopting an "go in the direction of flow" attitude is a win-win situation when it comes to fighting being overloaded by the stress.

Instead of imagining yourself as a rock solid and resilient in the face of every challenge you confront, think of yourself as a river, continuously and towards the direction you're supposed to go, regardless of any pebbles that life might toss at you. Keep in mind that a rock, no matter how strong, may break down under sufficient stress... however, the stream continues to flow and its waters move around the debris that comes in its way. The rock might be strong but it's not without its limitations andonce it is broken can't get put together. The stream however is able to adapt to changes in its environment and its structure, staying fluid, and moving on towards its ultimate destination. It is equally important that be flexible in your actions and thoughts in order to adapt to any stress that your life might bring.

Chapter 3: Limiting Beliefs Are The Most Often Cited Cause Of Stress

What beliefs are the most restrictive?
Beliefs that are restrictive are ones that make us feel a certain way to perform certain tasks. Because of our beliefs, it is only when I begin to believe I'm not enough. It's not possible for me to accomplish this. This isn't meant for me.
The beliefs that limit us are usually about self-identity and identity. These beliefs could also pertain to others and the world at large.
In any event they define the limits for us to follow.
The first step is to determine the beliefs that limit you. Many will claim that this is hard. This isn't the case.
It's a matter of figuring out in what areas of your life you're being restricted to the point of being ineffective:
What are the reasons you'd like to perform something but you can't do it, regardless of the reason?

Where would you like to stay clear of doing something however, you must do it for any reason?

If you reach a certain level of limit, there's usually some belief that is the limit.

Then, you must find the root of the limiting idea.

It's also a lot simpler than you imagine and does not require much contemplation or soul-searching.

Beliefs are shaped as follows If X is X, then Y, which is Z

For instance, "If I try, I'll fail. That is a sign that I'm a failure"

Then go back to the issues you noticed in the initial section.

If you were to do something that you would never normally do What would occur?

This is the 'if X , then Y'.

Then, think about what the implications would be in the event of such an incident.

This will give you the 'which is Z.

Then, you have to "challenge" the limitation or ask someone else to take on the task for you.

Luckily, there are general patterns that help bring about change in a restrictive belief. Two of them are:

(i) Counter-example

Limiting beliefs are formed from instances. If you are able to provide valid examples that do not lead to a limiting belief it is possible to make them aware of their surroundings.

You'll require a variety of counter-examples that work, as one example 'proves that it's the case'. A number of exceptions prove that the notion is not true and needs clarification.

(ii) Exaggerate

Sometimes, a very compelling counter-example can be the difference between success and failure and you are at ease to overstate your argument:

"All dogs are frightening? So is Scooby Doo?"

If you can convince people to laugh about their issues then you're already on the way to change their behavior.

Note: If you are challenging an individual's belief system make sure you are as gentle and gentle as possible. This is about the underlying principles of their beliefs here.

To summarise:

The beliefs that limit you can be simple to recognize and define.

After you've done that, you'll frequently see what you have in order to get them to fall down. the cracks will start to appear.

And then you can change them and redefine the limits while doing it.

We all have faith in New Year's resolutions and vows to one another. It's our inability to maintain them that makes us fall short.

The mainstream media pundits claim that simply introducing people to concepts is enough to break mental, or even belief limitations. The majority of the population who are not educated is convinced, and they wonder why their lives resume to normal after a period of one to three months.

When I realized that I was harming my personal life by making my own choices I began to look for paid, and non-paid sources for that type of assistance. The paid help was effective and gave me a positive feeling that lasted for a while. The non-paid material was just the same. Every person's life revolves around the book they're currently reading. This is since the next moment of uncertainty, or anger or jealousy, anxiety or brain dumps are right in the next corner. After that, life is back to prior temp-buzz pathways.

This may sound absurd, but is bitter and damages lives. The life of a person is damaged when repeated disappointments in failure to make improvements results in resignation and all its bleak situations.

That was the real reason for many talented people from India, China, Japan in coming up with ways for people to be able to consistently independently without shaving their heads or living in a colony, and break the negative, and restrictive convictions.

There was progress and this led to the creation of a group in 1930, whose primary aim was peace in the world, and economic prosperity, by ensuring the individual's happiness. Here's a summary of the process, as well as some of the ideas that go behind the method.

The average person usually has greater potential to achieve great outcomes than they realize.

The biggest obstacles to people from being successful are emotional rather than cognitive blocks. If you are able to get expert therapy,, then the blockages are able to be eliminated in a systematic and effective way through combining therapy and the knowledge.

If you're not able to get expert treatment for your emotional issues however, you can make advance. You just need to seek assistance from a senior practitioner who has tried the approach described below.

Here's some mental aid.

1. You are special, as is everyone else.

Be aware of this and safeguard you from prejudices based on cultural or discrimination based on ethnicity.

2. There is more to you than yourself to be a living being, as does everyone else.

Be aware of this and ensure that you don't harm your relationshipsand the environment.

3. There are things you're aware of and many you don't. This is true for everyone.

This will help keep you from feeling unworthy.

4. Nothing happens unless the conditions are met.

This knowledge aids in understanding the origins of.

5. What goes around comes around.

This one sentence will keep you from making wrong assumptions about what to do.

6. Life is constantly changing, but LIFE continues to flow.

This powerful piece of wisdom can help ease the discomfort of impermanence.

7. We don't need to be 100% at Whatever We Do

It might seem obvious however, I was raised with strict middle-class Indian parents with one wish for me - that I would have a better future than what they had. To help make this dream real I had to meet their high expectations of me in any tasks I took on. It was art competitions, dance classes martial arts classes, or school exams, I was required to succeed in every single one of them. If I failed, they'd be able to clearly state how disappointed they were with my performance and how badly I not done my best.

These expectations remained with me throughout my adulthood and led me to conclude that regardless of what I did in my life, I needed to be successful.

Don't get me wrong. Ambition isn't bad.

However, a desire to be successful at everything to the point that you are flooded with guilt and self-recrimination each time you fall short is not just harmful to your mental well-being, but also to your physical and emotional health as well.

A failure in a tiny project which doesn't really have any impact in the overall plan of things could bring your confidence down and cause you to feel that you're not adequate enough.

If you fail in one endeavor, you're in fact a failure.

The truth is you're not.

Each person has strengths and weaknesses. given the time you're given on this planet the best thing that you could do is to play to your strengths.

Any efforts that don't produce tangible results, put them aside. Focus on the things that you excel at, and improve until you're the best at what you do than you.

For all the reasons, no one would like to be the old saying -- "Jack of all trades master of none."

8.Making mistakes doesn't make us A Bad Person

You're only a human. It is time to stop blaming your self for the moment you screwed up. I'm sure that you caused harm to you and others but it wasn't at your control. You did everything you could in the circumstances that you were in. You shouldn't be blamed for collateral injury.

You are able to let yourself forgive yourself. Self-love and guilt will harm no one and will do nothing to you.

Nobody is perfect every all the time. There is no reason to be ashamed of their mistakes, as they're no longer able to rectify.

Breathe, go on then let your past remain what it is. It's not yours to control and your future is. Don't be embarrassed by that one error you made in the absence of knowing more.

9. Spending money on experiences or things We Like Doesn't Mean We aren't able to save Money

My family wasn't exactly wealthy. Dining out and taking trips were rare as kids were always instructed to conserve as much money as they could. In the end, we utilized our pencils and erasers until the very last millimeter and wore our clothes until they were ripped or worn out, and we never demanded anything that wasn't necessary.

The belief was ingrained in me , even when I was an adult.

In college, I lived at the minimum, and never regretting it. However, when I began working I remember this moment when a group of colleagues planned a long weekend excursion to a hill station nearby.

My instinctive reaction was to respond "No" without knowing the reason I'd resisted.

I could afford the money and time needed for travel, however then, I was wondering why I did not follow the idea?

In a split second when I was in the middle, I realized the moment I realized that everything came back to my mental state. It was my habit to save every cent I could that allowing myself small pleasures was as if I was committing a crime.

The process of relearning this lesson was most difficult part, however, through time and repetition, I was able to get over it.

If you're similar to me, then I'll say that you don't need to feel guilty for spending money on experiences and things that make you feel happy.

You are able to buy that beautiful wedding gown that you've were eyeing for months. You're entitled to take the 14-day vacation in Tuscany with your loved one. A few little pleasures is not a sin when you do it in a responsible manner.

Keep a savings account. Learn about personal finances (or employ experts). Make sure you have a separate amount to cover emergencies. You are also free to spend the remainder of the funds on any interests you'd like to.

10. Being Fun Doesn't Mean We aren't responsible

You can have a break. You can invest your time and energy to things that fill you with joy. Even if your parents had to work so hard that they never got time to relax does not mean that you should be treated the same.

The idea of burning yourself out and working until you're dead isn't the only way to financial success.

Make time for yourself. Breathe. Enjoy a pastime or anything else that can make your chest feel lighter.

However, when you do this, make sure you don't overdo it.

Make a plan for your day in advance to ensure that even after your chores are completed you still have time for self-care.

Keep a notebook and write down your top priorities during the week. You should make sure to allocate some time for yourself.

Prioritise self-care. Get that set of fragrant candles you're worried will cause you to look unprofessional when you go to the cashier. Take advantage of a professional massage. Lay down, apply the face mask and close your eyes and then relax.

You're allowed for breaks. But, this does not mean that you're doing something wrong or aren't realizing your full potential.

You're being you. And at times, that's all you have to do.

11. Sexual desire is not shameful.

India is a nation of 1.3 billion people, and has zero sexual education. Through my entire life, the only thing my mother ever taught me was that sex is a sin and that I must stay away from it until I'm married. My virginity is precious and should be protected and only give it to my husband and not any other person. If I do not do this, no one will ever want me and I'd have to die on my own.

I was just a teenager. In my ignorance I was a believer, I had accepted this notion.

Now, fast forward to the time when I met my first boyfriend in college. He was a guy who the two of them wanted to be intimate. My brain said no but my body wanted it. I needed to exert an incredible amount of self-control, and then make him turn down.

Even so after a night of being on my own in bed, I was overwhelmed by feelings of shame and guilt. I was near to giving all of it to him. What could make me reckless to desire something that is so sinister? How can I betray my parents and potential husband in this manner?

It took years of changing my brain to be able to connect my beliefs with the desires of my body. If you've been conditioned to think in the same way as I did and you are a victim of this, here is a message for you: regardless of what the world has convinced you that your desires for your body aren't necessarily negative. The desire for pleasure is an opportunity to celebrate the chaos and madness one is as human being. Refraining from doing so is like telling the universe that you do not want to be a part of the riches it has freely given to you.

12. Intimacy doesn't have to lead to Heartbreak

Many of us have had unpleasant moments in the past when we had given all of our love effort, time and energy to a single person but they would later deny the gift and leave us in the midst of self-pity, and a ruined dream.

The relationships fail and, usually, there's no way to stop the relationship.

You can let a relationship that has failed define your love.

John was a fraud and an cheater. This doesn't mean that everyone is liars or cheaters. Sally was with a man throughout the time and you didn't even know it. This doesn't mean that all women have backup options available and can leave anytime you don't offer them the "fair bargain".

If you'd like to feel the joy of love for yourself it is essential to keep your heart open to find it and embracing it. The construction of walls around you to guard your heart will just cause you to miss the many wonderful people around the world that may be waiting around the next turn.

The world is filled with wonderful, loving people and you can be a part of attracting them. Don't be afraid to let your heart open due to a failed love affair. You have the power to control your love life the moment you decide to be loved and loved. No one and nothing will stop you from loving and being loved.

13. Being honest about being sad and tired, or sick Doesn't mean we're weak.

Another disadvantage of being a child in an upper-middle class Indian home is seeing your parents grow exhausted, yet keep an upbeat attitude "for for the good of their family". My father was always at work every day, regardless of how exhausted he was. My mom cooked three meals for the family of four every day, every day even when she felt sick. The sight of my parents working all day long etched this message into my mind that work is of the absolute importance. Anybody who avoids work is insecure.

However, in reality it's not.

You can skip your work if you're sick. You are allowed to change plans when you're exhausted. You can seek help if you're sick.

Being aware of your strengths is a great thing. However, acknowledging your weaknesses, accepting them, and then adjusting your life to accommodate it is more satisfying.

The ideas discussed in this article are derived from decades of research by a variety of brilliant individuals. They are renowned all over the worldin a dispersed and scattered forms. Simply knowing that you are aware of, comprehending and agreeing to the principles will not alter much beneath the surface of your mind-heart.The application of this technique is not going to accomplish the things you want to accomplish. It will help you improve.

Chapter 4: Watching What You Eat

It is also possible to reduce stress by being mindful of how you take your food. Certain eating habits can only serve to make stress issues more severe. You can stop that from occurring by:

1: Avoiding Sugary Foods

If you indulge in something sweet it is likely that you will have fewer physical manifestations of stress. This could be the reason as per Harvard Medical School - you are likely to crave sweets when you're stressed out and "stress eating".

However, researchers have discovered that over the long term eating a diet high in sugar could cause inflammation in the part of your brain known as the hippocampus. This can result in physical signs of stress. Psychology Today also reports that excessive consumption of sugar is associated with depression.

Additionally, eating sweet foods could trigger glucose spikes throughout your body. This results in increasing your mood. However, this spike quickly is reduced because the body produces insulin in order to regulate the sugar levels and your mood changes to one of being "low." The mood swings can cause symptoms that are similar to those caused by stress, or even worsen in the event that they are present.

Instead of hurrying to eat food items that are loaded with sugar decide to eat foods such as proteins and whole grain carbohydrates, fruit and vegetables. If you choose to do that you'll be improving your stress levels more rather than the opposite.

2: Avoiding Alcohol Or Caffeine

Caffeine and alcohol are among the most popular legal substances across the globe. Indeed, many take advantage of caffeine and alcohol to manage stress. But, using the drugs when stressed could exacerbate the signs.

Let us look at caffeine first. Caffeine is a well-known stimulant. It affects your body through activating the body's "fight or fight or flight" response. If your body is aware of the threat of stress it triggers the "fight or flight" response that's activated. This means that if you drink coffee when you're stressed it is increasing the stress issue more severe.

Alcohol On contrary, alters the balance of hormones in your body. It affects the glands that make hormones, as well as the tissues affected by those hormones. When your body's hormone balance is altered, it's unable to deal with stress in a way that is more efficient.

Alcohol also induces cortisol's release. As you've probably guessed that this hormone can aggravate the effects of stress.

So, if you're looking to manage your stress levels, it's important to limit your consumption, or refrain from drinking the use of caffeine or alcohol.

3: Follow a Healthy Diet

Beyond that it is possible to be a good person and stick to an energizing diet.

It is a largely ignored aspect of the ongoing battle against stress, particularly in light of the hectic schedules we have to keep these days. But, don't do not ignore it and you'll be at risk.

Doctor. Mathew J. Kuchan , Ph.D. says that an energizing diet can help build solid foundations for your body to protect itself from stress. The doctor further says that a balanced diet can reduce inflammation and oxidation. This helps to combat stress.

What's even more fascinating is that a healthy diet aids in blood flow. If blood flow increases within the brain area, tension levels are significantly reduced.

There is no way I can spend my time explaining how to make healthy eating plans because that's not within the scope of this book. However, there's a wealth of information on the internet that could assist you in figuring out.

Chapter 5: Strategies To Manage Your Thoughts To Control Anxiety

Anxiety can trigger physical symptoms such as a rapid heart rate and sweaty hands. It may cause you to restrict your activities and cause you to struggle to achieve an incredible most.

A healthy mindset can help you to prevent or manage discomfort.

Negative thoughts can cause anxiety or fear.

*CBT is a type of therapy that will help to overcome negative feelings with specific, positive ones.

The process of changing your mind is a process that takes time. You must practice sound reasoning every day. As time passes, your good reasoning will be able to work effortlessly for you.

Healthy thinking might not be enough to aid some people suffering from anxiety and stress. Contact your primary mindfulness doctor or advisor if you require additional help.

How can you use your healthy thinking techniques to help you cope with anxiety?

Stop and pay attention to your thoughts.

The first step is to recognize and put an end to negative thoughts, or "self-talk." Self-talk is when you contemplate about yourself and the experiences. It's like an journal in your head. Your self-talk could be objective and tolerant. On the other hand, it may be negative and unsupportive.

Find out more regarding your concerns

The next step is to determine if your thoughts are helpful or not. Check what you're saying to yourself. Does the evidence support the negative belief? Some of your self-talk could be true. However, on the other hand it may be half-detailed but it's been you have distorted it.

One of the best ways to determine if you're overly stressed about is to look at the probabilities. What are the probabilities or probabilities of the thing you're stressing about could happen? If you're a candidate for a job audit that contains a tiny review among a myriad of compliments What are the odds that you're at danger of losing your job? It is likely to be low.

There are several kinds of irrational thoughts. Here are a few varieties to look out for:

*Sharing the negative This is the time referred to as the process of sifting. It is the process of focusing on the positive and put the spotlight on the bad. Model: "I get so apprehensive talking openly. I realize that people are thinking about how bad I am in my speaking." The truth is that probably no one is more focused on your presentation than you. You might be looking for evidence that positive events took place following one of your presentations. Did people beg you to come back just a few minutes later? Did anyone tell them that you had done an outstanding job?

*Should: Every occasionally are prone to thinking about the way they "should" do things. If you find yourself thinking that someone else "should," "should," or "need to" achieve some thing, then you could cause yourself to feel awful. Example: "I must be in control at all times or I'll be unable to change to the circumstances." The reality: There's nothing wrong having some authority over what you manage. However you could create anxiety by stressing over issues you cannot be in control of.

*Overgeneralizing: This means applying one model and saying it's true for all situations. Look up words like "never" or "consistently."

Examples: "I'll never feel typical. I am constantly stressed out about everything." Realistically, you stress over a variety of things. But, really you are stressed about everything? Do you think you might be not telling the truth? Despite the fact that you might be stressed over various things, you might find yourself feeling calm and peaceful about other aspects.

*All-or-nothing Thinking Also known as "dark or white" reasoning. The model: "On the off chance that I can't locate the most appropriate line of work audit, then I'll be fired." The reality is that most execution surveys contain some helpful analysis, which you can work to make better. In the event that you receive five positive comments and a useful suggestion this is an acceptable survey. It doesn't mean you're at risk of losing your job.

*Catastrophic thinking is acknowledging that something terrifying thing could happen. This kind of absurd reasoning typically includes "imagine the scenario in which" is a question. Example: "I've been having cerebral discomforts lately. I'm stressed to the max. You should think about the possibility that it's brain tumors?" Realistically, if you experience numerous migraines, you must see a doctor. However, there's a good chance that this is a more common occurrence and less real. You may need glasses. It is possible that you have an infection of the sinus. You may be experiencing tension-related headaches due to pressure.

Select your ideas

The next step is to pick an accommodating alternative to the unhelpful one.

Keep a journal of your thoughts is possibly the best way to stop making notes, and deciding your thoughts. It helps you be aware of the self-talk you engage in. Write down any negative or negative ideas you've encountered during the day. In the event that you think you won't remember them at the end of the day, make sure you keep an eraser with you to record every thought that occurs. In the meantime, you can record supportive messages to confront negative thoughts.

If you keep doing this consistently and consistently, your precise, positive thoughts will eventually come out effortlessly for you.

But, there could be some validity in your negative thoughts. There may be some things to address. In the event that you weren't able to execute the way you would like on something, keep a record of this. It is possible to look at an arrangement to remedy or fix the issue.

Methods to calm Your Nervous Mind

Anxious thoughts can take over your mind and cause you to struggle to decide on a decision and then make a decision to deal with whatever problem is bothering you. Stress can also trigger thoughts that are too much, making you more anxious and leads to more thinking and more overthinking. How can you get rid of the endless cycle? Resolving your thoughts about the edge isn't going to work. They will just come back every now and then, with greater force. But, there are increasingly effective methods that you can gain from mindfulness-based pressure reduction and CBT.

The next article will provide 9 ways to help you to unblock yourself and move forward:

1. Try Cognitive Distancing

Try to view your thoughts as speculations, not absolute facts. Your mind is trying to safeguard you by anticipating the possibility of what might happen, but considering that something could happen does not necessarily mean it will. Check out the target proof What is the probability that the negative outcome could actually occur? Do you think there is anything positive that could occur? What's more, what do you believe is in the process of happening given your past involvement as well as other information you've gathered about the situation?

2. Then try Cognitive De-Fusion

Stop letting your thoughts get caught up in your thoughts. Imagine your thoughts as information that is moving through your brain. This is in contrast to the actual truth of an event. Our brains are very sensitive to danger and risk since it was the way we were able to keep our predecessors alive in the natural world. Some of your thoughts could be merely to create a molded response by a mind built for endurance. Decide whether you want to accept these thoughts, instead of simply allowing them.

3. Practice Mindfulness

Try to observe your thoughts instead of reacting accordingly. Consider your thoughts as mists that float across the air. Which ones entice you, and which are the ones that make you want to leave? Are there ways to unwind and just sit back and observe your thoughts rather than reacting?

4. Focus on Direct Experience

Your mind is able to create stories about who you are, what your personal identity is, as well as about your happiness and your cuteness. These stories are not always accurate. Sometimes, our minds are influenced by past experiences that have been negative. What are you doing currently? Are you aware of something that is actually happening or could happen? It is important to note that they're not very similar even though your brain might perceive them as a similarity.

5. Label Things

Mark the type of thoughts you're having rather than looking at its content. Be aware of your thoughts, and if you come across a judgement (e.g. how fortunate or unlucky the situation is) Feel free to label it as judgment. If you notice a stress (e.g. or that you'll fall down or suffer a mishap) label it as worrying. If you're constantly examining yourself, mark the process as criticizing. This takes you free from the demanding nature of your thoughts and helps you gain a better understanding of your mental processes. Do you want to spend your time judging and worrying? Are there more non-judgmental or stressed methods to view the situation?

6. Keep Focused on the Present

Are you letting your mind wander to the past? Just because something bad happened in the past doesn't mean that it has to be repeated in the present. Find out if the circumstances or your perception and capacity to adapt, have changed from the previous time. As an adult you are able to make more decisions regarding who you want to communicate with and a greater capacity to comprehend, accept or exit from an abysmal situation, than when you were a child or an adolescent.

7. Widen Your View

It's safe to say that you're focusing only on the most dangerous parts of an incident instead of looking at the whole scene? Unease causes our brains to agree and focus on the immediate risk without considering the bigger picture. Does this situation really be as important as your anxiety claims it is? Are you able to be mindful about this issue be the same in 5 to 10 years? If is not the case, then take a step back from the pressure.

8. Get Moving and Start Moving

Being stressed out about an issue and not having an answer will not help you take a more mindful view of the problem. This could in all likelihood reduce your motivation to take action by keeping your discomfort. When your thoughts are stuck in circles, you may disrupt it by moving about or performing some other task or activity. When you sit down, it is important to be able to see a different perspective.

9. Determine if a Thought is Beneficial

The fact that an idea is true does not mean it's beneficial to focus on it--at all times not necessarily. If just one of ten applicants will be able to get the position you are looking to get, and you keep looking at the possibilities it is possible that you will end up being discouraged and will do not even think about applying. This is an example of an idea which is true, but is not a good one. Focus on what you can use and then let go of the rest!

How to manage your Activities to reduce anxiety

I experienced one "ah ha" moment about one year ago that totally changed my life. Maybe it's the insight I've had of my life.

As with a large number of people I was busy, distracted, and engaged. I was shuffled around with a plethora of balls all around without gap... two little children, a business and a house to manage and a charitable endeavor to complete and tennis, as well as my Bunco gathering, and Book Club, without any conclusion to be seen. I would start my day with a brisk pace and then go to bed at 12 pm, with just half of my plans for the day firmly in place. "One week from now , things would settle down" I'd tell myself only to discover that the next week was just as busy. I was always anticipating the day when things would slow down however that date didn't show up.

Sound natural? I'm sure it does due to how I seldom encounter people who aren't overly stressed and overwhelmed by the task of completing all of the tasks.

Our society is a hectic and exhausted society. In addition, I've been enticed by the notion that being occupied is good - it means I'm productive and not lethargic. I've even gotten myself into the habit of boasting (camouflaged as wailing) about my being busy to others. Every now and then I'd take on an uninvolved game with someone to determine who was the "busiest." That's crazy!

We don't get decorations for destroying ourselves - we simply get depleted!

It struck me one day. My life is full and, more importantly, it's full. I'm completing many things I have to complete in light of their ability to are enjoyable and fit into my plan. Instead of declaring, "I have a truly busy week "I started replacing "occupied" by "full" and then, all of a sudden my perspective changed. I'm an "entire weekend." I live an "full existence". It is filled with exercises that benefit my family, provide me with motivation, inspire me, and are a delight.

This may appear to be an insignificant and simple action. However, changing one word has also altered my perception of the world which is quite powerful! I began to make an objective decision to see the beauty in my life. I realized that I was blessed to be able to enjoy such a large number of opportunities to meet, connect, and have encounters. I realized that I'd rather not to sit and stare at the television or munching on bonbons (in all likelihood, most of the time). I want a life that is full that is filled with love, joy and happiness.

I realized that everything I do is a choice. I select the people I surround myself with as well as the activities that I do in my day. It is then my job to decide on the right choices and be sure I'm picking activities that I am happy with and not just to keep me entertained.

Then I started to look closer and when I saw something that wasn't a good fit and didn't feel "full" for me, I decided that to let go of that item. As time went on, I was able to say "no" to things that didn't satisfy me. When I am beginning to worry about my schedule, I know that I am blessed to have accomplished a huge amount of things that I am proud of.

The effects of anxiety can impact your mind, body and behavior. Here are some suggestions for managing anxiety through the management of these three areas.

I suggest you pick the ones that seem to be the most important to you.

A healthy body

The physical symptoms of anxiety may include muscle strain, a fast heart, a twitching, perspiration and breath slurriness. They can occur in a flash and cause a lot of stress. They can be anticipated or diminished by self-reflective practices and winding.

1. You must take care of yourself.

Consume standard, well-balanced meals (for instance, three healthy meals every day).

Limit or avoid alcohol or nicotine admission.

Regularly exercise, particularly with the cardiovascular aspect or unwinding.

Engage in self-mindfulness as a habit - such as, for example, relaxing exercises or regular breaks.

Have a decent rest schedule.

2. Breathe.

Breathing well can slow down or impede the uncomfortable response, and provide the impression of peace setting, unwinding, or establishing.

Relax and practice your mind for a single moment whenever you're waiting on something (for instance, holding in line in anticipation of a test that is about to begin in the event that you are stopped at a traffic signal).

Try extending your exhalation, or outward breath. Take in for four seconds, then exhale and exhale for five or six seconds. Try this for at least a few minutes each throughout the day, or at whatever moment you feel it's appropriate.

3: Be mindful

The ability to observe our body and environment with a calm and non-judgmental approach will lessen feelings of nervousness and help to create a sense of calm.

Relax your eyes. observe your breathing. You can see the shape of what your body is doing, feel how intake of air feels, and what sensations you observe.

Focus your attention on the sounds you see, smell and the sensation of contact with nature around your body.

Switch your attention between your body and your surroundings for a few times.

4. Use cues to Relax

When you realize you're feeling in tension or you feel you're unable to release anxiety or stress, use this as a trigger to practice rehearsing the unwinding process in more standard ways.

Try fixing and discharging various muscle groups, and work on loosening the ones that tend to be tight.

Imagine that when you breathe in that any tension in your body is leaking outward. As you breathe in, imagine that it being replaced by energy, vitality, and peace.

Imagine a scene or scene that's unraveling for you imagine this when you are feeling stressed or anxious.

Make time for normal unwinding and enjoyable exercises, such as massage, steaming showers exercise, or simply going out in nature.

Mind healthy and happy

Anxiety is often accompanied with mental actions that are distracting, irritating and unproductive. This can be a result of stress or distracting yourself with worries or negative outcomes. The more you are stressed the more likely it is likely to occur.

5. Be Realist

Often, when people are anxious they consider the most shockingly awful outcome to their situation regardless of whether it will likely not occur. This creates anxiety and its ramifications.

Be aware of your situation or your signs.

Remember that emotions aren't real regardless of the fact that you're afraid of an outcome, does not cause it to occur or cause your stress to work out.

Use rational thinking - try to consider a potential outcome or outcome that is not too cataclysmic, but more likely to occur as a general principle. It is possible to ask for assistance from others at the beginning. Keep a record of your reaction for an update for the future.

Consider instances when your worries were rebutted.

6 7: Interrupt Anxious Thinking

It is sometimes difficult to make coherent arguments especially when anxiety is present. The brief interruption of your thoughts can help you discover your reasoning and choose what you'd like to pay attention to.

Find out if you are experiencing constant and unpredictable stress is the case "if" being a believer is a problem for you.

Explore some unique (and absurd) methods to impede this destructive process Take, for instance,

Sing your frustrations to a tune that is completely absurd, or speak them out into a fun animation voice.

Choose a captivating idea to focus on or think about, for instance something you're planning or you are happy with doing.

You can listen to music or read record a book. Remind yourself of the work you're doing by telling yourself that stress isn't helpful.

7: Control Your Stress

If stress is hard to manage, takes you away from your day to day tasks, and stretches your thinking, consider various strategies to reduce stress and allow yourself some time.

Find out if the strain is within your range (includes an angle that is within you control) or is not solvable (outside that of your reach).

Utilize critical thinking to focus on the reasonable stress. It is essential to clearly identify the problem and think about possible arrangements. make use of experts and con leans to select the most effective solution(s) and then create an activity plan to tackle the problem.

To deal with unsolvable stress, try unwinding or other techniques to limit your negative response to the circumstances.

Be mindful of your thoughts and only once. Use the stress diary or journal to record your stress every day (up to 20 minutes). If and when those stressors come back in the course of the day, inform yourself that you've just been stressed out about that day.

Imagine a space that is empty to keep your stress in - imagine you placing your stress in this, and then naming them in the process, and after which you can rationally place them on top. Enjoy a calm thought or focus on the task you're working on.

Chapter 6: Your Lifetime Relaxation Techniques

One of the biggest issues with stress is it's difficult to know how to handle it. If you've ever been worried about something , and then started to feel anxious because you were unable to manage these anxiety, you'll know. But, there are numerous strategies you can apply to help manage your stress and let it go away. Learning about the various methods of relaxation, determining the ones that work best to you and incorporating them in your daily life when required is crucial to managing anxiety and stress and remaining in control. Relaxing and being able to take your mind off of things is important when encountering situations that result in your anxiety levels to increase and make you feel anxious. Relaxation techniques that are effective will help you manage your emotions and manage your emotions before they become worse.
Breathing Techniques
Deep breathing is among the most frequently used methods for people suffering from stress

levels that are high as well as anxiety or panic attacks. If you begin to feel your stress levels increase and you are feeling stressed, taking a few deep breaths is a great way to assess yourself and take control of the situation. By taking a moment to breathe deeply in and out can cause you to be distracted for a moment by taking your breath in instead of focusing on the issue that is worrying you.

Understanding what breathing techniques work best with you, and the best time to apply these techniques is essential to help to manage your anxiety levels and ensure that worry and stress do not overtake you when you are in stressful situations. A well-timed, steady breathing routine can be the most effective in gaining control of your thoughts and emotions in stressful situations. Inhaling deeply for four seconds before exhaling slowly for 4 seconds and then repeating until you begin to feel more relaxed, could be among the most simple techniques to practice in managing your anxiety. Breathing in through the nose creates a natural tension in the breathing and allow you to concentrate on breathing and remaining at peace, not focusing on what causes you to feel anxious and stressed.

Advanced Breathing Techniques

While deep breathing is something everyone can perform to calm themselves and restore their peace during stressful situations, occasionally higher levels of stress require more sophisticated and targeted breathing methods. This type of breathing technique is employed by yoga practitioners and even when meditating to in bringing peace to the mind and body.

Breathing through the nostrils: The breathing method is believed to bring peace and equilibrium, something you'll surely enjoy if you're especially stressed over a particular issue. Make sure you're comfortable in your posture prior to performing this breathing method as it requires concentration and stability. It is also known as Nadi Shodhana practice, you perform this breathing method by covering your right nostril using your thumb and breathing slowly through your left nose. As you inhale then open your right nostril, then over the left side, and exhale out of one nostril on your left. This is a fantastic breathing technique to use where you have to concentrate more, like during an exam or presentation.

Breathing techniques for the abdomen: With both hands on the top of your chest, and the other one on your stomach and breathe deeply via your nostrils until your diaphragm expands enough to create a stretch within the lung. Averaging between six and 10 of these breaths for around ten minutes each day can assist in reducing the heart rate and blood pressure. This is crucial for dealing with stress.

Conscious Relaxation

You may believe that you're at peace - maybe you're relaxing in a hot bath or relaxing on the sofa on a weekend, but there's an endless stream of thoughts going through your head. It's possible to ease our bodies into relaxation however when handling stress, it's crucial to try to calm your mind, too. Breathing techniques can aid in the process of relaxation because practicing them will force you to concentrate on your breathing and not think about other things that could cause you to feel stressed or be anxious. By focusing on your taking your breath in and making an conscious effort to relax will help you focus on thoughts that are spiralling out of control, and helps you get control of your anxiety.

One of the most effective methods to relax your physique and your mind is by practicing methods of relaxation that progress. To rid yourself of the most tension is possible, from your neck down to your toes you need to put your eyes shut and concentrate on tensing, then relax all of your muscles for a few seconds at a time. Begin with your toes and feet, and then work your way up, through your buttocks, knees and thighs as well as the stomach, chest muscles, arms, hands neck muscles, facial muscles and even around your eyes. When doing this, it's essential to keep taking steady, deep breaths. It can at first be difficult to stay focused and focus, so inhaling through the nose, and holding for five seconds and then releasing the breath slowly will assist. Keep in mind that if holding your breath feels uncomfortable, you should reduce the duration until it is something is easy to manage.

Chapter 7: Thinking Restructurally To Reduce Stress

One of the main reasons stress in people is due to the way they perceive. In the majority of cases people believe they are in a worse situation than it really is, which causes them to be stressed. For instance, after you've submitted your research report at the request of your employer, you don't expect him to mail it back to you since you believe that you put your all into this project. You're angry and frustrated because you believe that your boss isn't a fan of your efforts, or simply wants to show you a difficult time. Instead of stressing yourself out and dwelling on the negativity you're experiencing breathe deeply and take a look back and consider the real motives of your boss for reasons why the project was handed back to you. Is it because there's an opportunity to improve? Is there something you missed that you'll should revise? The way you organize your thoughts can help you overcome the habit of thinking reactively and reduce anxiety.

What are the reasons to restructure your thoughts? Because bad thoughts put you in a negative mood. This could affect the performance of your brain and reduce focus and also impact your relationships with other people.

Cognitive Restructuring

Retrospectively taking a step back in order to analyze the circumstances to develop a successful strategy is what experts refer to as cognitive restructuring. Psychologist Albert Ellis introduced this technique in the 1950s in order to deal with the negative thinking patterns and unhelpful behaviour. It's a well-tested method that allows people to be more conscious of their negative and reactive thoughts so they can "re-frame" the thought to be more precise and less stressful thoughts.

Cognitive restructuring is one component of Cognitive Behavioral Therapy that is employed to treat patients suffering from depression. Nowadays, this technique is also used for treating a range of mental illnesses like post-traumatic stress disorder or PTSD and addictions, phobias or chronic stress. A recent study found that this treatment method was able to help patients lessen the impact of extreme grief and trauma.

You may not be suffering from these kinds of mental health issues however, you are able to employ cognitive restructuring to reduce your anxiety.

Utilizing Cognitive Restructuring

For mental restructuring very first step you must do is to take a deep breath. It can be difficult to concentrate and evaluate the situation objectively when you are agitated and overwhelmed by emotions. Try breathing exercises or meditation to relax your nerves to enable you to look at things from an entirely different way. This will allow you to focus and become more objective when reviewing what you are thinking about and also the environment that you are currently in.

The next step to do is to analyze the circumstances. Keep a stress journal and note down the details of the event that led to you to think negative. After that, take a pause for a few minutes and then determine your mood. Note down your feelings in the moment; were you frustrated, angry or upset? I suggest that you express your feelings in one sentence to ensure that you are capable of discerning the distinction in your attitude and thoughts. (Moods can be described using one word, whereas thoughts can be described in several sentences.)

After you have analyzed your mood, the next step is to write down your thoughts immediately following the incident. A few examples to include are: "Maybe I'm not cut out for this position," "He's personally attacking me" or "I do not see any potential within this organization." The next step is to make two lists: write down evidence that backs your opinions in one as well as evidence that does not support your beliefs to the contrary. Make sure you are impartial when looking at the evidence, and don't allow your emotions to influence you. (ex. "My boss was able to identify the flaw within my document" (ex "The revisions aren't too significant and don't require any additional effort.")

After you're done review the two lists you've made and think about both sides of the issue. Develop a balanced understanding of the events that transpired and then write down your thoughts. (ex. "My report was excellent but I missed certain minor mistakes.") When you've done this, you'll realize how much your attitude has changed. All your negative thoughts and anger are gone because you decided to look at the situation in the first place. The last thing you must do is consider what you can do to fix the situation and whether you should act or not.

It can be difficult to implement cognitive restructuring initially However, after some time you'll discover that this approach is simple and efficient in helping you cope difficult situations.

Chapter 8: Sleeping Well-Being

Stress can affect length and quality of sleep. Lack of sleep and stress can have a significant impact on physical and psychological well-being. Experts suggest that you strive for 7 to 9 hours of sleep each night, depending on their age and other aspects. As per the Centers for Disease Control and Prevention (CDC), 35.2 percent of adults within the USA are getting less than 7 hours of sleep each night. This could lead to an insufficient amount of sleep that results in psychological and physical health problems. The research has shown that, however, the function of sleep isn't completely clear. It is a facilitator for a wide range of actions. This includes modifications of tasks and repair of muscles, for example, the process of immersion.

Sleep Deprivation and its Effects

The National Center on Sleep Disorders Research estimates that around 40 million Americans suffer from a sleep disorder. This includes a broad range of diseases and illnesses that include insomnia, sleep apnea or restless legs syndrome. The number of ailments is increasing and are causing a variety of disorders. People are experiencing problems at late at night and throughout the day related to sleep. Depression of weight gain and elevated blood pressure are merely some of the ailments that could be linked to the connection between stress and sleep as well as sleep . This could be a cyclical process. Stress can lead you to suffer from sleep-related physical and mental health problems that can lead to stress that causes sleeping less well at night. Understanding how stress and sleep can affect your life in reducing stress and get an understanding of the issue could enhance your wellbeing and health and, most importantly can contribute to better sleeping. Lack of sleep may result in a lack of energy as well as a general lack of energy and problems working. Sleep deficiency could cause effects in certain situations such as when there is someone operating machinery while exhausted. A night of rest is not likely to cause injury However, sleeping less can increase the risk of developing chronic health issues.

According to a report by the CDC the people who sleep under 7 hours sleep every night are at a greater risk of developing likelihood of developing these conditions:

Obesity
Heart disease
Diabetes
Stroke
Depression
arthritis
Kidney disorders

Although a variety of causes can trigger these conditions sleep deprivation can accelerate their growth.

The Link Between Stress and Sleep

Stress can have many meanings However, it's a response that's been evolved in both animals and humans in order to enable them to handle crucial or risky situations.

For people who suffer from ANS, the system may be affected through stress (ANS) in which hormones are released, like adrenaline and cortisol. These hormones cause blood to circulate through the heart to organs and muscles and prepare your body if required to take action. This is also called the answer. It was essential to survive. These days, it is possible to trigger the reaction -- issues at work or relationship issues.

What kind of stress can affect your System Over The Long-Term?

It's normal to feel overwhelmed however, chronic feelings of Stress can trigger the body to remain in an arousal state for prolonged durations. If you're suffering from this type of condition the health of the individual can be seriously impacted.1 Effect of stress is that it could cause sleep lack. Being in a state of alertness can trigger thoughts that occur at night , which can delay the time of sleep. Sleep can trigger stress. According to an National Sleep Foundation survey of people aged 13 to 64 due to stress in the past month. Stress Keeps You Up During the Night -- The Cycle of Sleep And Stress

There are a variety of ways that sleep can be created through changes. The adrenaline and heart rate can trigger development, and then shift along with a feeling of unease. The body believes it is experiencing stress. It's because it's not be sleeping , and therefore in a state of danger! There is a possibility to fall asleep , but not be able to stay asleep, and you could awake at night time. It might be difficult to get up and relax your thoughts. When you go to bed, you are worried about the relationship, job, finances or any other thing worries you. You are either working too much or having a lot to do during the day can cause stress and you may not have the time you need to rest and get to sleep. You might not be able to be able to sleep if you don't go because you've been working too hard and feel over-stimulated when you fall asleep. In the absence of time, at the at the end of the day, you forget the time to do an activity. A lot of stress on your schedule and inadequate time can mean you're not able to spend time with at home with friends and family or take wholesome and relaxing things that help relieve Stress which can lead to. After a poor night's sleep, it is possible that you will require caffeine to keep you awake and thereby bringing an unending cycle of. There are a few of ways that stress may affect sleeping quality and could keep you awake.

Reduce Stress Levels to Enhance Sleep

In reducing their stress levels, a large number of people can enhance the quality and duration of their sleep. There are some chronic sleep issues that might need medical intervention like sleep apnoea, insomnia In the event that you are experiencing sleep problems as caused by Stress There are strategies you can take to improve your sleep. Check out some of these techniques and tips and try incorporating a few to see if you can notice any changes in your sleep quality.

These lifestyle changes can aid in reducing Stress:

Mindfulness Meditation

Meditation is a way to make one conscious of their surroundings. The aim is to recognize the thoughts, feelings and feelings without responding to them, which takes place both within and outside of. Studies have revealed that this technique has numerous advantages. It was discovered that meditation can cause Stress depression, anxiety and anxiety. More research on whether or not mindfulness is a therapy however, it is an effective method for people.

The practice of mindfulness for 30 minutes can be an effective method to improve sleep and reduce stress.

Exercise

Physical exercise is an effective tool for improving well-being and wellness and also giving benefits. Research suggests that there is a positive benefits of exercise. Well-being in the mind can enable it to serve as a treatment for stress and related ailments. This can reduce the need for further treatments. A 2017 review found that physical exercise can help reduce the effects of stress and stress. There is evidence that exercising has a direct impact on your sleep quality for older adults with difficulties sleeping. Engaging in moderate exercise that is physically challenging, like running, can improve sleep quality and decrease stress levels.

Other Lifestyle Changes

The next lifestyle change could be able to help people lower their levels of stress:

Making the switch to a healthier lifestyle

Reducing the intake of caffeine and alcohol

Avoiding working from home and looking over work mails throughout the end of the day

In need of assistance from family members and friends

The process of reducing stress can be complicated. It's Vital to determine the source of Stress that is connected to a relationship or work. Although these issues may be slow and difficult to solve, eliminating the cause of stress is essential to get.

Enhance Your Exposure Daytime

If you work during the day at work or live in the northern hemisphere, it is possible that you will not be sleeping and your daytime routine could be affected. Research has shown that exposure to light sources in the indoor space during the day can help people sleep better in the night. A good daytime routine has been proven to decrease stress and depression. Make sure you are able to regulate your circadian rhythm. You will get plenty of sunlight, and if you can't, think about making the decision to stay for the entire day, with someone close by.

Try Some Pure Comfort and Health Methods

Meditation, Meditation, and other methods of relaxation have all been proven effective in treating sleep and stress-related disorders. There are many yoga and guided meditation patterns specifically designed for people who have trouble sleeping. Spend some time during your schedule to wind down when you are done with it. Even if it's just 10 minutes to do a short meditation before you go to bed, you could see an improvement.

Try aromatherapy

Perhaps incorporating the use of aromatherapy in your daily routine can assist you sleep. A study found that patients receiving intensive care who could not be sleeping had a higher high stress level and greater standard of sleeping.

There are numerous ways to make use of essential oils to aid in a better sleep and relaxation including the use of air diffusers and pillow sprays. Lavender and chamomile are two essential oils that have soothing properties. Bathe in a tub prior to sleeping or before bed. You will find an air diffuser next to the mattress to moisten the air and to infuse it with.

Make the Room An Den Of Zen

Relax and relax before going to bed. Do not bring work with you and choose to purchase linens in a variety of hues, like white and gray. Make sure your home is free of clutter and other sources of stress and keep separate devices from your bedroom and your medication. Create a schedule that will last with at least one hour, and continues until you try to put your head on the pillow.

Try journaling

You may be able to reduce stress prior to going to you go to bed. According to the University Of Rochester Medical Center affirms that journaling can help lower stress, deal with Stress and emotions and manage depression. This is true and can cause anxiety as you work through the issues currently creating Stress and could be used to monitor the stressors that you face every day, and this means you will be able to learn techniques.

Write Out Your Financial Statements

Sixty-five per cent of Americans are asleep. It's a lot easier said than done and tackling your financial issues could be an excellent way for ensuring you get an ideal night's rest and decreasing anxiety. Although it might not be simple to ease the financial strain, you might be struggling, as you'd been asleep, preventing your financial problems. And, as they don't "vanish," they At the thought of consolidating your financial debts could cause problems with your debt. in the near future, you should work to reduce the stress and make adjustments.

Take a look at nutritional supplements

Before you start taking sleeping pills, consider herbal supplements and nutritional remedies for sleep. Although all supplements for dietary use should be used under the guidance of tryptophan and melatonin by an expert, B12 and magnesium are just a few of the supplements that could help you, as well as herbal teas like valerian, passionflower, and lavender.

Fix Your Diet

In addition to ensuring you do adequate exercising, Diet is a significant component of the sleep/stress factor. Reduce your intake of caffeine throughout the time you get up, so that you're not keeping you alert. Avoid eating too late at night and ensure that your diet isn't loaded with sugar and carbohydrates that can affect the blood sugar as well as your energy level. Give your body a chance to rest and avoid snacking.

Get Expert Advice

If you are unable to find a solution and you've tried over all methods, you could benefit from the assistance of a sleep specialist. A sleep expert will attempt to figure out what's wrong with as the reason why you're not sleeping. If you've eliminated the possibility for apnoea or other sleep disorders, you can ask a sleep.

Sleeping habits can be used to monitor heart rateand breathing during your sleep and you can determine if the issue is stress-related or something else and making sure that you aren't suffering from an problem. Make sure you are in control of your health and study the ways that stress could be impacting your sleepand how your levels of stress are affected by the absence of sleep! Increased levels of stress can cause a variety of problems and ailments that can affect your health and well-being. When you understand what's going on in your body when you are under stress, you will be able to know how the best way to manage your body's entire structure, both inside as well as out, and learn how to modify or change your lifestyle and surroundings. If you apply two or more methods to manage Stress You could notice changes in the quality of your sleep and overall health.

Chapter 9: Learning Positive Attitude Tips To Declutter Your Mind

Imagine for a moment that you have an artist gallery. The walls display some of your most loved paintings you've collected during decades of collecting and exploring, the ones which have truly impressed and inspired you most out of all the paintings of paintings you've seen.

The mere act of entering the main room, with artwork that are displayed in a variety of ways will bring the viewer to what art can do and how it can enrich your life in a way that is unlike anything else. It is also an experience.

The best way to boost your creativity and get you off to your own creative space to grow.

It sounds like a wonderful scenario, doesn't you think? However the gallery where the paintings aren't displayed in a way that is clear. They're usually covered with old furnitureand massive electronic devices that haven't seen electrons flowing through their veins for the past. There's debris and dust all over the place, and there's barely a space that is hip-width wide winds through the entire area.

The stunning and possibly charming gallery looks more like a backyard with the bizarre light of shade that comes from an artwork trying to peek through the chaos.

We often think we'll get rid of clutter in our homes in the new year. We want neater closets and more organized systems, as well as the living space that is truly an feng shui. We want the places that we live in and work in to be efficient so that we can achieve more and feel better.

Think of your mind as a separate space in your home, asking you to organize and clearing out. Our minds

are the kitchens that fuel our jobs and also our collaborations. Spend a few minutes to look over your head. What is it like? Do you see objects scattered all over the place or is there through the path that leads to your destination? It is said that the National Science Federation has, in actual fact estimated that humans produce anywhere from 12,000 to 50k concepts every day. In his blog article, Emotional Wholeness, Dr. Deepak Chopra mentions a clinical research study that has pushed the amount to 65,000! It's easy to understand the way that a large number of thoughts can create a amount of chaos. How many of those ideas are unimportant or even unfavorable?

We have the tools to gain the attention of our ideas and also implementing an orders. Many successful individuals already know their process. Personally, I believe that inflow of thoughts is a proven method, as is the effectiveness of mind clarity.

What do blood circulation and its effects mean to you? What does it feel like? Do you have a picture of it? Since there are only a little time in the day to accomplish what is already to be completed, de-cluttering the mind can be incredibly beneficial for us during our daily tasks , allowing us to achieve greater efficiency in the tasks we undertake. It's easy to notice the negative impact from stress in our daily lives. The process of de-cluttering provides you with time to concentrate on you and also provides you with the time to gather ideas . It will also assist you to keep a straight line between work and along with parenting.

If you're interested in sitting still more than exercise, then it's an excellent instrument for you. The practice of meditation is pre-dated by the majority of world religions. Hindu scriptures dating back more than 5,000 years reveal the very first method of reflection taped. Since meditation has actually gained appeal among our overwhelmed generation, educational books and courses are just only a click or just a phone call just a phone call away. I meditate every day. It is recommended to begin this practice in the event that you do not already practice it. Even just five minutes every day can be beneficial to your health. When I first began to meditate I was told not to try to do more than two minutes at a time. For me, the most beautiful aspect that reflection offers is the simplicity. Sit at a comfortable spot with your eyes closed and allow your mind to drift by.

If you sit quietly, you'll be able to see ideas coming up within your head, similar to clouds that form against blue sky. Instead of trying to decode your thoughts, let each of them go while you concentrate on the clear blue sky in your mind. If you can unleash each cloud with confidence your mind's clarity is increasing and you become more effective in all you undertake. Whatever your method to clear your mind, it isn't difficult ... similar to as arranging your stack of shoes in the floor in your wardrobe!

The importance of removing mental Clutter

The constant stream of thoughts, worries or information to keep in your mind: all add up to a psychological chaos. What would you be able to accomplish when all your mental space was cleared? Are you present and focused or are you working through your list of business, thinking about the emails that you have to reply to, or deciding what to eat for lunch and also trying to catch up on your online reading (like the book I mentioned, for example)?

These thoughts could be causing you to lose track of your focus and advancement. It's what we call a mental chaos. The majority of us get up early in the morning and look at our phones to check our emails, texts and news swirl inside our heads before we brush our teeth.

The car's oil needs a change, your kids require haircuts and the dog has to get his teeth cleaned by the vet. Do you have a shopping list? Oh, and do you remember that blog comment that you read yesterday? Perhaps you didn't notice it. Maybe you should reconsider and erase your comment. There's also that task at handWill it be completed in time? Is it going to be a success?

We're thinking about the past, and we're worrying on the future and not letting administrative issues overshadow the most important thoughts. We allow digital distractions to enter and try to accomplish everything at once. This isn't functioning. These items take up a lot of space in our heads and there's not much room for the tasks you're supposed to be doing in developing a revolutionary app or writing the best selling book.

The psychological clutter takes us away from our current situation and out of the work we're juggling and people we work with.

What if all that mental space were cleared?

What if we decided to pay attention to our choices? What if we began taking a look at the diversions we are avoiding and sifting some of the sludge out?

What if we decided to conquer that mental chaos? What can we do from that space of our minds, or, perhaps?

Here's how we'd go about it:

We'd have better clarity in our thinking and focused.

We'd become more efficient, and we will have more room to come up with imaginative ideas. We'd be less stressed and less likely to lose particulars.

We'd be more restful without the nagging which makes us stay awake.

We can focus on the important work instead of

getting distracted from the details.

It might not be simple however, regardless of the method you decide to use to get rid of the mental clutter The results will be absolutely worthy of the time and effort. Imagine a world in which

Every person was less fearful and more relaxed, happier and more productive. What are we putting off?

Working: We must to manage the entire view of a task

It is important to keep all the information in your mind, instead of being focused on only one thing at a moment while we change between tasks. It helps to focus and also as increases determination, which, will allow you to get more accomplished.

Maybe for you, it's electronic distractions that have created confusion in your mind. The devices that disrupt our focus hinder you from being focused on your job and objectives. If this is the case for you, which is the case for most of us, then it might be time to try some new electronic routines.

The opposite from an emotional mess transparency. Focusing on and developing systems can help you develop and implement to-do lists , so you'll be more productive.

The simple strategies such as this can help you to clear your mind without getting overwhelmed by the task at hand.

In the home In the house: Believe it or not physical clutter can affect your brain as well. If your home is in dirty, clearing the space could be the first step in clearing your mind. You can go one step further and clean the mental clutter just as you do to clear your physical clutter. If you want to live an enjoyable home life the ability to take a long-winded brain dump is a crucial ability to master even if it does have a different name.

Just like no two products are able to be in the exact same location in the

Your house your home, there are no two ideas that will share the same place in your head. Take note of the thoughts you dwell on. Consider how these ideas may be affecting your life and the people who are around you. Make a wise choice.

The Soul of Yourself: Maybe you're a minimalist as you're working or your home What do you think of minimalism as a way to improve your life? We absorb a lot of things every day that we require a daily routine to clear our minds. One type of clutter is interruptions. You can, however, learn to identify the things that distract you from the goal you're trying to achieve. It is possible to make conscious decisions on whether you want to allow these distractions enter your life.

We may not be able to see it and see it, but that doesn't cause a mental mess to be any less stressful. Our minds can be used for more than to-do-list storage. What can you accomplish when you put aside the mess and learned to be completely present?

10 Tips To Clear Your Mind

Everyone has to deal with it. In some areas of the world, we are confronted with it, whether in our closets, our workplaces, or within our bodies. Most distracting and chaotic area is our minds. The water is running, or the stove running. Unable to find words, struggling to articulate a point. If we're absorbed in our thoughts, lost in worry it's hard to be clear or at a zen moment. If we're not in a clear mind we lose connection to our surroundings, ourselves and the people in our lives. A mental mess can throw us off-center, disrupting our equilibrium. It's so chaotic and disorganized that we can get confused.

Cleaning Clutter at the Basis Personally, for me, it was a relief to know that I was raised in a large, loving family. However, a large family can be a home to all sorts of junk. Growing up by four siblings sharing a bathroom, one TV and a phone Let's just say that it became a bit sour. It was certainly not helping the fact that Mom was a shopper, and Dad was an avid packrat. The fear of being claustrophobic in my childhood led me to want to be clutter-free. It wasn't until I was in my time in college, far from home that I realized that my thoughts were the primary source of all the mess I carried around Absolutely nothing and no one else was responsible. After a major quarter-life crisis, it became apparent how I was jeopardizing my own peace and equilibrium by bringing my head-trash with me-- the junk I kept up in the upstairs.

Then I decided to purge my home of clutter starting at the bottom of all things--my mind.

How can you begin clearing the mess you don't even be able to see? The process of decluttering your mind requires us to be aware of where we place our focus and the way we use our time and energy.

Just like the stacks of papers that surround us, we collect many thoughts in our brains every day.

In addition to the physical clutter surrounding us, our constant interactions with technology and endless mental to-do lists create an unnoticed ball of twisting threads in our brains. We are stressed and are unable to focus or make the right decisions. Instead of looking inward and employing holistic methods to relax our minds our first choice is drinks or comfort foods to unwind and relax.

Do you recognize that? It is true that cleaning the mind is an ongoing effort and the consistency of your efforts is crucial in maintaining a certain degree of cleanness up there. To clear away the cobwebs and perform some soul-searching it is essential to conduct some major decluttering and compartmentalization of your brain. These are the ten actions you could follow to discover your inner tranquility (and maintain it!).

1. Get rid of your physical clutter

It's not a secret that physical clutter adds to the psychological and mental chaos. It may be impacting your brain in greater ways than you imagine when you're constantly seeing a sign of chaos from out of the corner of your eyes. It's a constant thing that you'll feel an increase in tensioneven if it's only a littlebut then you'll be more stressed by the pressure of having to tackle the issue.

Take it slowly. Take care of your problem areas or areas where you are spending hours inat the very least, you should create an organized and tidy space where you can unwind and unwind each day. Don't limit yourself to sprucing up your personal space. Your email inbox as well as social media could use some spring cleaning, too!

We believe that it's vital for your mind to follow this 9 week Happy Body Formula program has an entire week dedicated to decluttering with specific tasks for each day.

2. START A JOURNAL

We at Happy Body Formula, we are big fans of journaling. The benefits that have been proven for writing things down is extensive and a more organized mind is among the most persuasive arguments. It's a thing that's available to everyone and there aren't strict and sluggish rules to it. All you need is a pen and notebook.

Bullet journaling is an amazing method to start. It involves list-making as well as short-chaining thoughts. This is a great option for people who are scared of starting a journal, particularly those who aren't writers. It is a way to keep track of the schedule of your social and professional obligations such as calendars, food sleep and exercise logs, and many more. It becomes addictive once you start making lists! This is among many of the simplest and efficient ways to see what's going on in your mind. Also, once it's written printed on paper, it may not be as difficult to write it down.

3. GET OUTSIDE

Outdoor activities are calming for a variety of reasons. Most of us spend the majority of our time indoors. If you take a moment to think about it, you could find yourself noticing the amount of time you're spending outdoors.

The majority of the time people are outdoors is due to work. For example walking to and back to the station, walking with your dog, or getting and returning your vehicle to work or home.

Instead, think about incorporating more outdoor time that is planned into your schedule if that your mind's clutter is getting out of hand. If you're looking to increase your "cleaning tasks," get some exercise when you're out and about.

Outdoor running, trekking or kayaking, and other similar activities that aid in relaxing and gaining views as you work up a sweat and release your positive brain chemicals. Being immersed in vast landscapes is a great way to help us feel our worries small amount smaller and more manageable. Likewise, a nature stroll can help us focus on other aspects (i.e. instructions, bird sounds different types of trees) and also help get us away from our thoughts.

4. DITCH THE TELEVISION

Television can be a an annoyance however, it's a guilt-free pleasure for a lot of us. With services like Netflix is now easier than ever to binge watch ... And you'll know that it's not over until Season 1. If you're struggling to make time to take care of yourself, or any other suggestions we've listed in our 'clear your mind list for today cutting back on some of your time watching TV at night can help you clear the space for an hour (or three!).

Although television appears to be an excellent way to unwind the mind and ease tension however, it's actually doing the exact opposite. You're exposed to constant changes in other people's opinions, thoughts and opinions that in turn affect our own thoughts.

It's not easy even if it's unconscious. If you're still not sure to get rid of your TV restricting your media consumption of websites that you check outis an great option. This is done by setting time limits for the amount of time you spend with your electronic devices or what gadgets you use on a daily basis or both.

5. DO NOT MINIMALIST

The most difficult part of clearing out clutter is to keep your mind in autopilot. Your mind should be kept at a level that is manageable of chaos in all instances or, in the ideal case, with no stress!

Some people may be a good idea to reduce. Think about the huge amount of things we must deal with and consider each day. Imagine if you could remove a handful of items completely, instead of trying to control the tension?

We're easily by the notion that our happiness will improve when we gain more. We're however convinced that things work quite the opposite direction.

Minimalism requires you to think about what you truly require and would like to have.

If you're dealing with material matters or just wandering

Thoughts, this elimination process will bring your mind some important positive things. Additionally, it will enable you to make a decision the things that are necessary and positive in your daily life.

6. Stop Overbooking Yourself

We live in a frantic society, for the most part. We're constantly shackled by long and sometimes unattainable lists of things to do in addition to social obligations! We overlook the fact that we have the ability to simply say "No" which is why we give in, even though we really don't have time to do half of it.

The mere thought of all this can stifle your mind and stop you from doing all that you would in the beginning - which leads to the tendency to feel stressed.

If you're trying to clean your thoughts, make a promise to make a few fewer changes. We're insisting that skipping some is fine, especially when it means your peace of mind is at the chance of being ruined.

Be realistic about what you must do in comparison to what you'd like to accomplish, and make sure you reserve the time for yourself first. Sometimes an adjustment in your mindset could be all that's needed. Even if you reduce your expectations in your lifestyle, you'll not lose out on anything that is truly vital to you.

Chapter 10: Relaxation Techniques

The majority of us today think that relaxing means sitting watching television or watching a movie , playing video games or something similar. While these types of activities can be beneficial in other ways however, they are not able to minimize the negative consequences of stress. Relaxation methods that reduce stress stimulate and trigger the body's natural response to relaxation. The techniques for stress-fighting relaxation include deep breathing, meditation yoga, rhythmic exercise and more.

What is the best way to combat Stress?

Relaxation techniques like meditation, deep breathing, etc. trigger the natural relaxation responses within our bodies by activating the following responses:

* Slower heart rate
* Deeper and slower breathing
* Stabilization or drop in blood pressure
• Relaxation and relaxation of the muscles
* An increase in blood flow to the brain

The body's natural responses caused through relaxation techniques counteract the negative effects of stress like an increase in heart rate, more rapid breathing, increased contracting of muscles, and decreased circulation into the brain. Alongside countering those negative impacts of stress practising relaxation techniques can help in increasing your motivation and energy levels. Here are some efficient methods for relaxation and stress management that you can practice at your home.

Breathing via the Diaphragm

We breathe in and out without thinking about the possibility that the moment this aspect of our lives slows down and we die, then we are dead. However, the reverse is also true that if we're dead this means that we are unable to breathe. The breath and the life are incredibly interconnected with one another. We think of breathing as something we do for a living.

The diaphragm is the organ that we breathe through. often called abdominal breathing - is the way we were designed to absorb and release air. If you look at the breath of a child through the diaphragm, you can observe their stomach moving upwards and downwards. The pressures of modern living have forced us to breathe through our chests, and the majority of us aren't conscious of our nature of breathing through the diaphragm instead of the chest.

In times of stress the chest tightens and breathing becomes shallow and slow that triggers the fight or flight response that is required to survive under stress. Even in modern times, where survival stress isn't an problem, we still utilize this same method. It is essential to break this habit while fighting modern-day stress-induced emotions.

* Sit or lie down in a comfortable place

Place one hand on your stomach, and the other hand over your chest.

* Breathe through your mouth.

Now, breathe slowly through your nose while maintaining your chest in a still position and expanding your abdomen.

* You should feel your abdomen contracting and expanding when you exhale and inhale and exhale, while your chest is unmoved.

Try this relaxation method on a regular basis for around 20-30 minutes.

Breathing through alternate Nostrils

This breathing technique is inspired by the ancient practice of Yoga that was practiced by thousands of people of years in India. Indian subcontinent. Breathing in alternate nostrils can lower stress and anxiety, can lower blood pressure and enhance cognitive abilities. Below are some steps to take:

* Relax in a comfortable spot, in a quiet, uninvolved place.
* Use your forefinger , or thumb to close one nostril.
* Breathe in through an open nostril, and count to five.
* Now, shut the nostril in this direction and exhale by the other nostril, which was shut previously.
* Repeat the process beginning with the opposite nostril, each time.
* You may practice this meditation at any time.

Meditation

Meditation is an ancient and most effective relaxation techniques for stress management. Meditation boosts your resilience and helping you become more calm in stressful situations. Research has proven that meditation can increase the production of fewer neurons in the amygdala, which is located close to the brain, and is that are associated with stress, anxiety and anxiety.

Meditation aids in the increase production of GABA which is also known as gamma-aminobutyric acids, a neurotransmitter which aids in relaxing the mind. GABA can reduce brain activity and allows you to feel less stressed and more calm. Meditation can help you quiet your mind and allow you to be in control of your negative thoughts, which are the reason for stress. Meditation can help you stay in the present being aware of all the wonderful things you can enjoy by turning your attention off things that are uncontrollable, like worrying about the future or regrets of the past.

The most effective method of meditation to aid in the process relaxation is one that assists you concentrate on your mindfulness. Here are some mindfulness methods of meditation that you can implement into your everyday life:

The meditation of Mindful Breathing I Below are some steps to mindfulness breathing:
* Sit comfortably in a quiet place
* Close your eyes.
* Breathe normally, but do not attempt to alter your breathing pattern.

Take a moment to notice how your breath passes through your nostrils.
* You can exhale and inhale every when you breathe out, and breathe in, for your mind concentrate in your breathing.

If a thought pops up to mind, you can observe it, mark it, and then bring your thoughts back to your breath.

The method is easy. The key is to persist with your efforts. The purpose of mindfulness meditation isn't to get rid of thoughts, which isn't possible. It is important to be aware of every thought that occurs and to find the ability to eliminate it once you have acknowledged it. The purpose for mindfulness practice is to force your mind to concentrate on one thing, which is the breath. In this instance, it is your breath.

Mindful breathing meditation II This is a different method of meditation that focuses on your breath. The steps are as follows to follow:

* Sit in a comfortable position in a quiet spot
* Keep your spine erect but comfortable
* Restart breathing normally
* Now, take a moment to count your exhalations and inhalations.
* One exhalation, one inhalation
* Then, two exhalations Two exhalations

Repeat this procedure until you've reached ten breaths and 10 exhalations

Once you have completed one, begin with the next set starting from one

Repeat this procedure for around 5 times

Once you've completed the series of repetitions, take a deep breath normally and slowly let go of the contemplative state. There will be thoughts that are likely to arise. Pay attention to each thought, note it, and then go back to counting your breath. Gradually and with regular practice, you'll be able to master this method and gain the benefits.

A Body-Scan-Meditation - this method is great for relaxing your whole body and mind prior to sleeping. Through meditating on each aspect of your body you'll be able to free yourself from knots you have never seen through conscious awareness only and nothing more. Being aware of a knot can be enough frequently to let go of the knot. This can help you ease into a more relaxed state and help you fall to a restful, deep sleep. Below are some steps you should follow to complete a body scan meditation

* Lay down in a comfortable place
* Take some time to discover your normal relaxed, tranquil and steady breathing pattern Now, concentrate on your body
* Concentrate on each area starting with the left toes and moving until the left hip and

then through the left foot, ankle the knee, calf and thigh.

If you discover knots that are not conscious in your body, breathe deeply into the knot and feel knots being released , and that particular area becoming at ease

Repeat this on the other side , too.

* Then, concentrate on the hip, followed by the chest, stomach and the head region.

* In each location you go, let loose any knots in your anxiety by focusing your attention and using your breath.

Focus on your palms, arms and your fingers, feeling the stress that has built up in your body by the fingertips of your fingers

Meditation via Guided Imagery

It is a powerful method to decrease anxiety and stress through the use of visualization and imagery. Furthermore, guided imagery techniques are employed to enhance performance and meet the goals and targets that are set for you. The techniques of guided imagery are utilized in the following scenarios to improve results:

* For treating depression and anxiety disorders

* To improve immunity

* For treating high blood pressure

* To help with pain management
* To improve sleep
* To manage stress

Be sure to follow the following tips:

* Close your eyes.
* Imagine a tranquil and serene location
* Represent it as clearly as you can.

Concentrate on the things you hear, feel as well as feel, taste and smell

It is vital that you include all your sense organs and sensory systems into the experience.

* For instance If you're picturing the sunset over the beach:
* Watch the sun set on the horizon's far side, casting its orange and red lights across the skies
* LISTEN to the seagulls and the other birds' chirping
* SMELL the earthy smell of the ocean
* Feel the waves crashing your feet
* Smell the salty air

Let your worries and tension melt off your body while you imagine these images of peace and tranquility. While you wander around this tranquil space, allow your brain to be absorbed by the feeling of tranquility you envision and envision a happy location. After you're done close your eyes, and slowly come back in the present. Enjoy a few moments of the blissful end result of this meditation practice.

It is crucial to keep in mind that all types of breathing techniques and meditation require time to master. When you are in your beginning days, which may be as long as a couple of months, or even more You will be awed by thoughts that are not related. Each time a thought comes into your head, take note of it, mark it as a simple thought. Then refrain from responding to it or react to it, and then let it fade away from your thoughts. Remind yourself to the meditation.

Chapter 11: Make Care Of Yourself And Be Happy Every Minute Of Your Life

You are in need of affection, love in addition to your attention most. If you do not give yourself these, you'll be emotional overwhelmed. To take care of your daily chores, feel productive and make the most of your energy, time and effort in the most efficient possible way, you must take care of yourself.

Here are some essential items that many of us overlook and then complain about our fatigue. Implement these simple suggestions and activities into your routine and you'll be amazed at how calm, physically fit and emotionally content you are.

#17: Work on Your Diet

Your diet plays a crucial part in determining your mood and well-being. If your diet is comprised primarily of processed, packaged and junk food that is loaded with trans-fats as well as Genetically altered organisms (GMOs) as well as processed sugar and salt, and other artificial ingredients and that's the reason you feel tired unmotivated, slow and tired. These foods can upset your hormonal balance and health.

Slowly replace these food items with fresh vegetables, fruits organic, whole wheat products. They provide healthy nutrition, including carbohydrates, protein, good nutrients, fats, minerals and fiber. All of these will keep you healthy.

In addition, you can add eggs and citrus fruits, fatty fish such as avocados, berries, and avocados to your daily diet. These are all rich in B-complex vitamins and omega-3 fatty acids and antioxidants that enhance your mood, decrease the stress you feel, increase your immune system, and provide you with the energy needed to attend to your tasks effectively.

#18: Get Sleep. Well

The scientific evidence suggests that for optimal functioning adults require the same amount of rest every night, throughout the day. If you're sleeping between 3 to 5 hours a day it could be one of the causes that you feel grumpy, tired, and angry often.

Give some consideration to your mind and body and give it adequate sleep every day. Apart from the exhaustion caused by sleep deprivation, you rest for longer than you should and sleeping insufficiently impacts your brain health as well as overall cognitive function.

When you are asleep the brain filters important information from irrelevant fragments and stores crucial memories. This process begins when you fall into a deep slumber that is approximately four hours after your first night's sleep. If you sleep only for between 4 and five hoursor so, then your brain does not have sufficient time to think about and preserve memories. As a result, you're likely to be in a state of forgetfulness throughout the day.

Begin to sleep well by establishing a set time for bed and a morning routine. Get to bed an hour before the time you normally go to bed and take part in a relaxing task like reading an ebook or listening to soothing music. These activities can help you relax and allow you to fall asleep with a degree of ease. It is also possible to take the time to soak in a warm tub to soothe your nerves and help you rest better.

You should wake up the same time each day, even when you were unable to sleep at night. By sticking to your sleeping and wake-up times for a few weeks will gradually manage the cycle of circadian (brain's internal timer) and you'll begin to fall asleep in the evening.

#19: Increase your Heart Rate up

If you lead a slow-paced life that is characterized by only a minimal amount of exercise, this is yet another reason why stress is a regular feature of your life. Move around and get moving, as physical exercise increases the production of positive hormones within your body. These hormones include dopamine as well as serotonin and both can improve your mood. In addition, exercising lowers the levels of cortisol within your body, which helps to fight stress more effectively.

Begin by performing routine chores and walk as often as you can. Gradually, you can engage in vigorous physical activities every day for 15 minutes and gradually build up a habit of doing it. You can practice swimming, yoga, aerobics in a brisk stroll, run or engage in any sport that is active. The goal is to keep your heart rate to a point that you feel happy and content. As time passes, you can you can increase your workout time to 30-40 mins and then stick with it throughout your life.

#20 20: Do Things You Like

If you don't take the time for activities that fill you with joy and happiness, then you're not being kind to yourself. That's why you feel irritable and dull.

Write down the kinds of things you love doing and make sure you do them often. It is possible to participate in at least one each day, and then create a variety of different routines for your week.

Mondays might be 'walking in the park ' days Tuesdays might be 'taco nights' Wednesdays might be "warm bath days" and other days. This way you'll take care of yourself every day and feel great about your self.

21: Love Yourself More

Furthermore, and as a matter important, you should be more loving of yourself. Be kind to yourself, acknowledge your strengths more, recognize your achievements, and accept yourself for the mistakes you made and setbacks.

Being kind to yourself will help you to get through life rather than wallowing over the mistakes you made as well as painful moments. This also helps you radiate joy to everyone around you. When you see other people smiling for your positive attitude, you'll feel more relaxed and less anxious.

Chapter 12: Control And Management Of Stress

How can we handle stress? How can we deal with challenges and how can us turn ourselves into medical assistance without causing more stress? It isn't it stressful to admit that we require medical treatment due to our body's inability to cope with stress? There are many ways to manage stress, starting with simple time management all the way up for seeking medical help. Every day, we are faced with different types of stressor is similar to playing a game. And as with any game, there's an winner and a loser. Whoever wins will reflect the way people handle stress. Prior to birth, the obligation to manage stress is upon the mothers. Smoking cigarettes during pregnancy can to relieve herself, smoking can ease her emotional stress as well as that of a child, but is not the health stressor that causes the impact of smoking to children. The most effective way to manage stress for babies in during the birth is to deal with the mother's stress. Every stage of life has its own method of dealing with or managing stress. However, generally the most commonly used are as follows:

immediate Family and Friends. It's important to recognize that we are all a human beings and we are not able to manage all things. It's just that simple. It's not a fairytale to be living, but a constant battle to live. Keep in mind that no one is an island and we must find strength in a person. This is the reason why friends were created They are the person who we can seek out in times of happiness and battle.

A child may not have the capacity to deal with challenges or things in life however, with the help of parents, everything can be dealt with and children can comprehend. In times of stress teenagers do not seek out the assistance of an immediate mother, but rather of friends. Because the adult's ego tells them contrary most of the time they'll need their own an adult companion who can help them face the realities of their lives.

Medical Aid. Stress and other toxins in our body can make us weak and prone to illness. This is the reason the importance of science and medicine in controlling stress is crucially required. Stress that is chronic needs medical attention because your body is unable to anymore handle the stress, and neither can alternative therapies. Don't hesitate to seek advice from medical professionals and experts based on your needs. Chronic stress is a matter of the use of science and human skills to manage. The effects of depression are real, and may cause death if not addressed. Although we are blessed with relatives and friends who provide immediate relief from depression, the problem is that stress is a major issue when someone is in a lonely place.

The initial sign of stress occurs in your central nervous system. This is which is the one that regulates your brain and the command to your body. A high-functioning nervous system can be harmful the heartbeat continues to increase and that will also affect the organs in your body. It is possible to experience frequent vomiting, frequent urination, muscular pain and headaches as well as other. Stress can also weaken your immune system . This can result in illnesses and weaken your antibodies against other diseases. Accept that there are aspects of the world that science will resolve, and chronic stress is one of to be addressed.

Finding Inner Strength - The body is able to heal itself. Take a look at how wounds heal itself. The body is protected by antibodies. our body from harming invaders. Antibodies can also be referred to as immunoglobulins, which are created through our immune system to keep bacteria, viruses and other chemicals from harming our body. Thus, we are able to fight the effects of stress within.

The psychological aspect of inner strength is what keeps you going and allows you to live your life. It is what makes you feel happy is a source of peace, and gives you that sense of security and safety. It may come from within and be bolstered by our emotional attachment. It's supposed to answer the question of what makes you feel happy and satisfied. It is possible to take a look at the things you do like dancing, swimming and singing, gardening and cooking. Activities that take you away from stress and puts you in a peaceful state. The majority of women find the benefits of massage and shopping as to relieve stress as effective. This is also where finding your interests starts, by finding what you're good at, discovering your passion and discovering your passion for art.

Strength in the inner part can be boosted by talking to your trusted friends and spending time with people who can make you feel safe. Strengthening your inner self will help you deal with the detrimental effects of stress on your body. Being passive at times can be beneficial so you won't be negatively affected, it shouldn't be done every day.

Ask Nature for help. It is a way to see the beauty of nature that makes you feel at peace and have that feeling of joy. As sour as it may sound, but a stunning flower can bring a smile. Every time you smile on your eyes, a celebration takes place within your brain. It releases hormones known as endorphins that can help soothe your nerve system. Relaxing your nervous system helps the body's system to work effectively and it may lower your blood pressure and heart rate.

The beauty of nature encompasses all creatures that live with it, which includes humans. However, let's focus on the benefits of having pets in the house, even the pet you have is snake. It is possible to talk to them and they'll listen, but don't expect them to respond. When you fail to do that, it is an indication that you need medical treatment.

Pets can be a source of happiness and also provide comfort.

Enhancing Faith. This involves using your religion and belief to combat and reduce the effects of stress. Be a part of your faith, whatever religion you follow sing their hymn and listen to their teachings. The essence of curing disease is beyond healing the physical body but rather of the soul and mind. Stress can intensify or speed up the symptoms of a specific medical condition, however the power of faith could be a great aid. One just has to trust in God.

Stress is a symptom of a disease, and it is a fatal condition. The funny thing about a condition is that it may enter our bodies like an emitted light however, it takes time and perseverance to end it.

Management and Handling of Stress

Every day with a variety of stressors, and as an activity, there's winners and losers. Whoever wins is a reflection of how an individual handles to manage their stress.

The world is as simple as the picture above. It's not a fairy tale that we be living, but a constant battle to make it through. It is not always easy on our own; we must be able to rely on another. That's is the reason why friends were created.

Inner strength is the thing that keeps you going and makes you live your life to the fullest. It is what makes you feel happy and calm and gives you that sense of security and safety.

It's not as corny as it sounds however, a gorgeous flower can cause a person to smile. When you smile on your eyes, a dance occurs within your brain. It releases hormones called endorphins that can help relax the nervous system. Relaxing your nervous system helps the body's system to work properly and it may lower your blood pressure and heart rate.

Keep your faith in regardless of your religion Sing their hymn and take in the lessons. The essence of treating a condition is not just the healing of the physical body, but also of the mind and soul.

Chapter 13: De-Stress Your Body, Mind And Soul

If you require an answer to your anxiety, it is important to adhere to the long-term strategies. For the most effective outcomes, you should practice these methods regularly.

Does it matter in the next year?

Always think about this whenever you are in a stress-zone. Whatever it is that you are worried about consider the impact it has in your own life. Your mental outlook is an important component of this. Whatever you believe in is able to make things come to life. Therefore, if you find something that doesn't matter over the course of a year then you need to decide to alter your current attitude.

Do you have a battle to win?

Most of the time, you are confronted with situations that don't matter to you, and aren't worth your time or effort. There are instances when you must put aside your worries and not worry too much. Make your choices wisely.

Don't let go:

What do other people think of your

A family member, friend or a friend creates trouble

If you face a rejection

If you make a mistake, it's a failure. (Is truly a failure even if you really took a chance and tried something? I'd say it's an accomplishment.)

Do not be a person-pleaser.

Beware of dressing, living eating, and doing anything in order to please others. If you put other people's opinions over your own then you will be overwhelmed. You are the only person you have! It's fine to tell "no" to things you don't enjoy. However, in reality, it's the perception of someone else's. Being nice to people usually leads to an internal conflict which is where you battle your own self. In order to relax concentrate on your own personal goals and utilize your uniqueness to bring joy and beauty to the world.

Start journaling

Journaling is a more effective method of creating a list of things to do. You can keep track of your daily, weekly and monthly tasks. Or just get your feelings out! If you record your plans, it is easier to prioritize and set aside time for things. You will avoid being overwhelmed, confused or from missing important deadlines.

It also tracks your spending, food moods, meals, and schedules for work. It's a lifesaver dealing with stress.

Declutter your life

There are a lot of unsolved issues in your life which pile up and cause chaos. There's many things to accomplish and so many tasks to consider that it can feel overwhelming. Similar to how you clear the mess in your home You must clean out your life too. Set aside time each day to look at how your life is progressing and what you can do to bring it back to a more balanced state. Schedule meetings, plan events and establish a schedule of calls for your children and/or family. The habit of following a schedule is beneficial when it comes to living a stress-free existence.

Physically fit

Similar to laughter therapy exercise releases endorphins into the body, which aid in decreasing stress. Spend time working to strengthen your physique. Engage in any activity such as running, walking, cycling or swimming, karate, aerobics, dance, cardio or jumping rope, for instance the one that is most suitable for you. There are many ways you can remain physically healthy, so pick the one that you enjoy and stick to it. It's entertaining!

You're not a juggler.

Set a time limit for an activity and make sure you don't overbook yourself. Scheduling your schedule can assist you in avoiding anxiety and avoid making too many plans. Every thing requires a certain period of time, and so it's important to know how ways to prioritize things. If you attempt to manage your plans, they don't come out well at the end you're feeling like a mess.

Set your boundaries clearly

A lot of times, stress is triggered when someone strays from our normal routine. Then, you'll be able to pop your "personal bubble." If a friend wants to talk about things you're not comfortable with, a person is too gentle with you or invades your privacy or violate your privacy. This happens in the event that you do not define your boundaries with a firm hand and people continue to violate boundaries. It is best to define your personal zone of comfort. Be specific about the things you enjoy and those you don't.

Try meditation and mindfulness.

Make time in your day, or at least a few times per week, to pay attention. When you wake up in the morning, as you get up from the bed, if it is possible spend 10 minutes to be in silence. You could sit outside on the patio, or even in your room, somewhere that is quiet. What are you grateful for? What are your dreams? What do you want to achieve? Simply, be quiet and get away from the noise and chaos that the world is known to cause to us. Just 10 minutes of meditation every day could result in the drastic reduction of the stress levels of your life.

Make plans in advance

If your week is hectic and puts you under lots of stress, set your agenda for the weekends. It is possible to prepare meals ahead or plan your outfits in advance and make quick hacks to clean to make your life simpler. Planning your weekends ahead helps to get through the work week by focusing on your goals and allows you to feel inspired instead of overwhelmed.

Make yourself ready for the unknown

If you are planning, writing or make a schedule in advance Don't be overly strict. Make sure you leave enough room for uncertainty , as nothing happens completely according to plan. If you are anticipating that there will be some uncertainty, you won't be as astonished by it.

Write a few lines down in your planner for the day.

Don't put things on hold to back, and leave certain time slots open to deal with the possibility of a delay or sudden change in plans.

Make sure you have a backup dinner ready in case anything is stale, or someone visits.

Always put aside a neatly ironed dressand save spares for managing your daily life.

Concentrate on the nutrition

Research has shown that when your body is fed properly as well as a healthy lifestyle, stress levels drop. Be sure to meet your daily nutritional requirements in terms of calories as well as vitamins and minerals. There are certain foods you can focus on that can help relieve stress. Here are some examples: Almonds, milk and oranges, spinach, oatmeal, salmon dark chocolate, and lavender tea.

Do a digital detox regularly

Don't be rushed in the mornings to respond to messages, like pages and upload images. Get your body up slowly and let your mind take in the events of the day. Begin your day by drinking the glass of water and keeping a journal. Go for a walk of 10 minutes out in the fresh air. Make a sketch or paint an idea. Explore a new and inspiring book. Prepare a delicious breakfast and sip your coffee in slippers! Set aside a certain time to use social media.

Join a group for stress management

There is no one who can comprehend more than people who have gone through similar circumstances. Join a club and get to know other like-minded individuals, which will assist you in creating an effective support system. You can gain about their struggles and become more knowledgeable about managing your personal anxiety. Additionally, watching someone else controlling their stress may inspire you and provide you with the motivation to be able to manage your own stress levels.

Keep it simple

Don't over complicate things. Be mindful of simplicity in your life. Simplicity and minimalism are inseparable. Make an effort to accomplish more in less time and maintain a the space clutter-free. Organise every part of your day. Make sure to break down complicated tasks into manageable steps and live life one day at a. If you adhere to an easy and simple routine you will be able to stick to it and feel satisfied!

Unwind, rewind and unwind

After each day, change the theme! Maybe you had a fantastic day and would like to take a moment to reflect on the day. Perhaps your day wasn't as planned and you'd like to get away. Be grateful for the good things that happened and feel grateful for it. Relax your body and mind to unwind. Engage yourself in the things you love doing like a hobby sports, a hobby or just spending time with your loved one. Always begin and end your day by establishing a calm routine.

Select the five strategies that resonate with you or that you'd like to test. Note these on the mirror or an adhesive notepad on your refrigerator, or wherever else you consider it to be the best place to keep you on track! It can take some time to make changes in your habits which is why you should take your time!

Chapter 14: Redirecting Stress To Good

Like a strong breeze the stress of life can be a potent factor that can trigger forward in radial ways, create a new direction, fight for rights and justice and stand up for the people you value. It allows people from different backgrounds to break up the debris or unite for a shared reason, or to promote political campaigns and boost business, break relationships, or join.

Let people have the opportunity to express themselves more than the things they normally are afraid of. Like tornadoes, the effect of stress particularly when it is accompanied by anger, could be disastrous

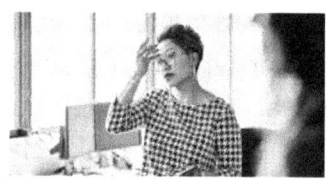

when left unchecked. So, if the powerful energy of anger or stress is pushed through you and not expressed or redirected by your internal energy, it is lost or shut off, just like the soda bottle shakes before opening. It is important to know how to manage stress by structures and directions so that its effects help the people around you instead of harming them.

Learn from our Ancestors

Traditional wisdom practices like Traditional Chinese Medicine (TCM), Buddhist philosophy and the Vedic system have emphasized the benefits of turning negative feelings into healthier and more vibrant ways over the course of hundreds of years. In the five elements of the TCM system anger, which is among the most destructive emotions, is viewed as a negative energy. It is linked with a liver that is not balanced stagnation, rapid growth, and leading roots to fall off the soil, and numerous health problems like hypertension, anxiety blood clots, and liver diseases. If it is in a positive balance the energy is able to communicate with compassion and the ability to feel compassion, strength rapidity of action, the ability to move, a gentle expansion, "branch" sound, spring color, and green.

The Vedic tradition, which dates back to 2000. C. in India The chakras system gives guidance on how to handle anger in a positive way.

Chakras, which translates to "wheel" (or "tornado" from Sanskrit are vortices that contain power and energy that rotate as the sun. There are seven major chakras within the body that are connected by the spine and each one is associated with distinct organs, psychological, physical emotional, and spiritual functions. They are also associated with the vibrations, colors, and sounds.

The chakra most associated with anger is called the 3rd chakra, which is that is located within the solar plexus. It's located between navel and the ribs and encompasses the abdomen, upper stomach, spleen the pancreas, liver, intestine and gallbladder. It is believed that this muscle center is a source of creativity and intuitive abilities as well as the intellectual aspect of the brain, which soaks into breaths, thoughts and experiences that allow you to identify yourself.

The 3rd chakra is the digestive tract that is healthy, where you can see the person you are feeding, what you consume and don't eat have the capacity to taking in and absorbing lifestyle information in a healthy way without becoming lost or misplaced. It is possible to let go and eliminate all things that do not benefit you, help you or help you. The chakra that is the 1/3 of unhealthy is marked by feelings of fear, insecurity and guilt, shame, anxiety, anger and numerous digestive issues. Be kind to you and with other people.

What does this mean?

He is aware that by controlling the stress response you can manage negative emotions. This can achieve through creating awareness and mindfulness through breathing techniques, implementing the practice of meditation communication with love, and staying fit. The ancient wisdom traditions encourage the application of these techniques not just to manage your responses to stress, but to transform the negative energy that comes from stress into positive energy that can benefit the person you are interacting with and other people. The main point is that these practices provide additional tools that will not only help reduce stress, but also redirect the energy to the positive side, which allows you to be productive. These tools don't include getting rid of stress energy and keep you occupied so that you can concentrate on your strengths and ultimately transform into the love of your life.

Make It Move to Release It

If you think about the way your body reacts during stress, you can feel it within your body or muscle like your energy has been impeded or stagnant. What can you do about the blockage of energy? It is to move it. The best method to release the energy block is by moving it, whether it's aerobic or movements that are performed during yoga, tai chior Qigong or progressive relaxation. It is also "displaced" by music, body or verbal activities, such as massage or Acupuncture.

Physical Exercise

Additionally, it is beneficial for your overall physical, mental or even physical health, it also helps you shed extra energy and release endorphins as well as other chemicals that can help you build an atmosphere. It can help you even when you're suffering from it. Think about running, stress or walking, biking or swimming when you're in trouble. You can dance, roll or play tennis, basketball or soccer. Training with weights is another alternative. Whatever you decide to do, take care, as you could get lost by your thoughts about negative things and you could avoid your form and injure yourself. Personally, I believe that physical exercise is an odd way to release my despair and anger. I also assist in slow movements, like the gentle forms of martial arts such as the form of qigong, tai chi, or even yoga, aiding in the creation of a feeling of calm and peace. This is what I refer to as meditation on the go.

Shake it Out

Begin to imagine things that are frustrating or unpleasant. Allow the stress to build and notice the places where you and your body feel restricted or confined.

Allow your hands and arms to slide to your side.

Begin to turn your legs around, beginning with your buttocks and then being and then the upper torso.

Join your arms together and shake them violently as you shake your head.

Your entire body shakes for about a minute as if you were getting rid of all the tension.

Outside

Be aware of how you feel.

Moving Meditation

If you don't get the luxury of heading to the gym or going to play in the outdoors and activities, you are able to perform stretching and rest exercises no matter where you happen to be. For instance, progressive muscle relaxation is a highly effective method that can alter the energy of stress and offer various yoga and breathing exercises. Particularly efficient are those that require turning the core of the body to neutralize the blockage of energy in the third chakra. Below are a range of exercises you could try. Pick one or try each one, in order, one after the other.

Supine Twist

Lay down on the back (on the floor, rug or grass).

Keep your knees close towards your chest, and then hold the knees in your hands, while breathing deeply and getting as close as you can to your chest.

Inhaling, allow your knees to slowly move to the left, while your head turns towards the right.

Breathe deeply , and after exhaling, pull your hip using your left hand, while your left arm extends out to the right.

Relax breathe and relax, stretch, and stretch.

Repeat this for ten times of breathing, one on each side.

Kundalini Kriya Pose

Cross-legged, sit on the floor.

Put your arms on shoulders, then use your fingers to run them over your shoulders.

Breathe deeply , then turn left.

Turn right, then turn left then slide it to your right.

Close your eyes and twist them twenty-six more times.

Alternate Breathing in the Nostril

Breathe deeply, then put your thumb on the right side and then press it down once you are able to exit your left nostril.

Your index finger should be placed on the left hole , and then raise your thumb to press the right nostril while breathing through the right nostril.

Your thumb should be pointing towards your right nostril. Lift the index finger off your left nostril. Breathe through your left nostril.

Repeat this process for 26 breath counts.

Sound Therapy

According to ancient beliefs various prayers and sounds may change the stress energy. It is possible to make these songs or sounds while you are paused or do not make any sound. The following exercises provide strategies I employ and find helpful.

"Shhhh"

According to the traditional Chinese medical practices, "sand" is a sound that soothes the liver.

Use your hands to make circular movements of your abdomen to ensure the liver is relaxed breathing. Exhale, and exhale again with your "shhhh" noise.

Place your hands over your stomach nine times while repeating "City."

Repetition "City" Nine times in your abdomen clockwise.

"Hello!" Shout "Hello!"

When you are sitting or standing in a position, you breathe deeply and exhale "Hey!"

Make sure you shout at least ten times.

"Ha!" With a slight movement

Place your feet on your shoulders.

Lift your arms over your head and take a deep breath. If you let your arm go and pull your arms upwards to let your body and head follow (so that you stretch your neck, and then slightly bend your buttocks) while shouting "Hey!"

Sing Loud

Find the song you like and take it off.

Sing at to the very top of your voice, and at the bottom of your abdomen.

Do it and dance along when you're doing this.

Journaling Stresses Out Stress

Writing down your thoughts and feelings could be extremely therapeutic and I highly recommend using a stress-relief journal, which contains reasons to write down that cause you to feel uncomfortable or anxious with all your feelings without taking a break or judging. This is my method I suggest:

Daily release of tension

Set a timer that runs for 15 minutes, or keep your eyes open.

On a separate piece of paper, separate from the other journals, list the reasons you're unhappy or annoyed and the things you feel you see, think or would like to do.

Do not let yourself be left out. Do not think too much about writing without filter. You can get it.

You can drag images or utilize simple adjectives or commas.

Make sure to stop the clock when it has shut off or you find yourself stuck.

Place your hands on the words that you wrote and repeat these words to yourself: "Now I will free me from my mind, body and my conscience."

Destruction of the paper by crushing crushing them.

Take a look at yourself the next day. If you notice that you're still unhappy or stressed the following day, do the same exercise.

Concentrate Your Power

Most of the time it's extremely difficult to stay still or quiet when you're stressed or talking about something about you're upset. Moving can help you shed this emptiness, so you can become more in touch with yourself, and manage your thoughts and emotions. One of the most effective ways to be on the land is to be in the natural world. Here are four easy activities to get you there. If you don't have the means to access to the natural world, these three sports are helpful.

The Nature of Centering

The aim of this exercise is to concentrate on the nature of mindfulness in order that you can use every conceivable sense to appreciate all the things around you having an illegal conscience and recognizing the relationship you share with the natural world.

Visit a place in nature you enjoy. It could be a forest or undeveloped field or beach, or your backyard.

You can relax and relaxed, lie down or take a position in the garden when you're at ease.

Stop when you close your eyes.

Take note of the sensation of air in your face.

Be aware of the sensation of air as you fill your nose, then your lung.

Be aware of the nature sounds all around you. Do you hear a song from a bird? Are the leaves moving according to the wind?

Be aware of the connection that your breath makes to breath, breeze, or the sounds.

Pay attention to the feel of the ground beneath your feet.

If you sit down, you'll feel the ground beneath you as you push it toward your hands and fingers.

Be aware of the soil, this is the type of land farmers are cultivating.

Enjoy the land and the opportunities it gives you.

Thank God for the nourishment provided by air, earth, sun and rain. Also, anything else that comes to your mind.

Be grateful for your place on earth, and also your position in between the heavens and the earth.

Breathe in deeply and slowly.

It is now time to start gardening using your mind take a stroll, or utilize all your senses to sit down or lie down and enjoy your connection to earth and heaven Listen to the world, listen as well as feel, smell and smell.

Rooting and Grounding

This is a modified version the qigong move (a version of slow and traditional martial arts) that requires you to move with balance and making use of your imagination to get there.

Keep your legs crossed over shoulder width, while keeping your knees bent slightly.

Maintain your chin straight Keep your chin straight, pull your head back.

Shut your eyes.

Take three or four deep breaths.

Pay attention to your feet's soles and then think about the connection between your feet to the ground.

Breathe in and imagine that you are putting the energy of earth onto your foot.

Inhale and release your energy from towards the back of your feet towards the floor.

Inhale deeply and then place your energy in the bottom of the foot.

Inhale, release your energy from to the side of your feet towards the ground.

Inhale deeply and draw the energy of the floor in the heel and then lean back, allowing your toes to show a little.

A cool exhalation and energy release emanating from the soles of your front foot to the floor. While lying on the heels of your back foot so that the heels can appear slightly. (Turn slightly every breath, and exhale).

As you imagine, the roots grow and then move deep into the earth, and connect you to the core of the earth.

Imagine that the root aids keep you balanced while allowing you to stay flexible and comfortable.

Breathe for at minimum 10 cycles, exhaling and inhaling and exhaling . Be sure to remain at peace.

If you're ready, get up. Be conscious of your connection to the earth, and consider what you feel.

Child's Pose

It is a form of yoga that's restful and healthy. It allows you to connect to the earth like the child in your life, so let it breathe slowly and exhale gradually.

Place your feet on the floor (preferably on mats, carpets, or grass that is soft).

Relax your shoulders and breathe deeply.

When you are done, walk forward and rest your forehead on the floor.

Keep it for at least five minutes for five minutes, and then breathe.

Liver smile

This is one of my most favored recognition exercises, which involves creating an inner smile to your coronary heart and your inner organs, specifically in this instance the liver, as well through the use of the sound associated with the balance of your liver.

Sit on a pillow or a chair with your feet. down on the floor, or on the ground, whichever more comfortable, and then shut your eyes.

Take three or more breaths, breathe in three counts, and then breathe in a count of five. Connect your backbone's bottom to the middle of your coronary heart as well as the highest point on your hair to the center of the earth.

Imagine that the electrical energy of the universe and earth connect to your heart when you exhale and inhale.

Smile and relax.

Smile while shifting your attention and focus back towards your heart. Smile with your heart. Smile, breathe and then breathe for five times.

When you are slowly focusing your attention at your liver which lies in the right rib cage take a deep breath, slow and deeply. Smile lovingly on your liver. Smile at your liver as you breathe in and exhale for five times.

Relax for five to ten minutes of breathing. You can say "show" every breath you exhale.

Take a moment to be quiet and notice what you feel.

Shift into Love

You've learned about the significance in love, and the healing power to improve your health and well-being I'm hoping you have enjoyed certain benefits from meditation. Since love can be difficult to attain in situations that are tense, it helps to shift the energy of stress to begin and then to focus on it. Once you are focused, you can change negative energy into something positive by using love by reviewing your IMT and determining how you could improve your self-care , or receive more help.

Be Careful

Your evaluation of IMT might indicate that you're irritable because of inactivity, lack of lack of sleep, loneliness, or anger. Therefore, you should first look at and revise the areas where you should apply love to your focus. You can create an overall plan (to relax, sleep or eat more nutritious food or eat healthier, etc.) and then plan your day to. And plan for the future "new program" might include getting massages or restoring your body, eating a nutritious meal, shopping for flowers for yourself or relaxing. Whatever you decide to do, be kind to yourself.

Social Support

The TMI test will reveal if you require additional assistance. You should ensure you have "Go" people you can call in times of need. They are the people you have identified, or plan to introduce into your life. People who are able to listen to your to you, cherish you or stay with you without trial. You'll be amazed at the number of people who could help you out when you tell them the things you would like them to accomplish. You could go to an emotional support group, counselor, therapist, or coach or connect with your loved ones who will remind you of how you appreciate them.

Help Someone Else

An effective way for redirecting and transforming your relief energy is to make use of it to help others, and not harming. Consider a reason you believe in the person and then make use of his stress to inspire him to help and love. If there's no reason for moving it, then you're able to assist anyone in need. Let go of your mind and your emotions and take a take a look around. Help an elderly person cross the street , or bring their food to home. Offer a hand to someone and smile. Help out in the soup kitchen. There are endless opportunities to volunteer in soup kitchens.

Chapter 15: Strategies To Effectively Deal With Changes And Obstacles In Life And At Work

Your life will be filled with challenges and changes. It's an inevitable fact. It doesn't matter if meet someone who always appears to be happy, they will surely have some awful tales to share.

The circumstances that cause the challenge or the change typically happen abruptly. Sometimes this can make it difficult to anticipate it. However, there are times that you are aware that it's approaching, and you are able to plan your preparations.

The arrival of a new baby into the household is an event you are able to prepare for up to a certain degree. It's not as easy to talk about falling on the stairs and breaking an ankle. Two distinct ways in which a change could take place.

The development of effective strategies for coping is your best choice when confronting challenges and change. The capacity to deal with challenges differs from one person to the next. This is why you may observe situations where certain people are praised for their ability to cope.

Resilience is a quality which determines your ability to can handle change or challenges and also stress. For the majority of people, they are working on this skill to achieve a state where they're not easily affected by changes. The majority of the time it's by implementing the appropriate methods.

If you're one of the people who keep trying to stay the course It is essential to alter your mindset. Since it will eventually take over and you will need to find ways to deal with. Strategies that you can employ are the ones I'll discuss in various parts of the chapter.

Practice Gratitude

There are many things to be thankful for in your life. Remembering these aspects will allow you to cope with changes. If you are able to practice gratitude, you'll be able be able to recall moments where you thought you would not be able to progress however you were able to.

These experiences can provide you with the inspiration you require to keep going whenever you are faced with new challenges

and shifts. If this is the first time you've taken this step there are a few things to be thankful for:
* Your family members
* Your health
* Your partner
• The reality that you've got an apartment
* The affection you receive from other people
* The lessons learned from previous mistakes
You should have enough funds to cover your requirements
* For your job
* For security and safety You can enjoy

Simply put any thing that makes you smile is something worth being thankful for. Keep these thoughts in mind when you face new obstacles and changes in your life.

Be aware of the things You Control

In every aspect of life, there's some limit to what that you can influence. If a situation turns into challenging or leads to the stress of a change, it's usually because the situation is out of your control. We are too focused on these situations that make it hard to overcome the situation.

In your personal life it is important to be able to accept obstacles and changes that you are not able to control. Focus on the things you are able to manage. They are areas in which your decisions determine the nature of your outcomes.

The loss of a beloved is a stressful and stressful event that is out of your control. It's normal to reflect on these incidents, and I'm certainly not saying that it's likely to be easy to make progress. In any case, you do not have the power to stop death or restore someone to life.

The quicker you can accept these realities that life has to offer, the more quickly you will be able to get your life back in order. This is the way it goes in all the situations we face. In the workplace, we complain about the character and attitude of our colleagues.

We frequently make it our task to force them to change. It is a way of focusing on something that is often impossible. If you don't feel the urge to do it from inside, you are blocking an immovable obstacle when you try to bring change.

You can evaluate the situation and identify factors you are able to manage. These are the opportunities to promote the growth of your life.

Find the Positives

The difficulties and changes your life encounters don't have been negative. There's always a positive aspect. It is important to look for these positive aspects.

Your struggles can help you become more efficient in how you manage money. It could also assist you in getting more connected to your loved ones members and encourage you to make new acquaintances. There is a chance of getting more assertive and creating more effective habits as you encounter the challenges or transitions.

While we may not like change but they can provide us with the opportunity to grow and become better individuals. With acceptance, you'll see how much improvement comes from the change and difficulties you face.

In focusing on the positives in your life, it's important to shield yourself from self-talk that is negative and thoughts. This happens when a changes or challenges bring about the possibility of a negative outcome within your personal life.

What you need to do to prevent negativity in your self is make sure you don't interpret any setbacks as a type of failure. This can hinder your ability to adopt positive thoughts.

The final reason you should take the initiative to seek positive things in life is because it isn't all roses. There will surely moments when it appears like everything is not getting your attention. Every action you take could be destined to go downhill.

This can lead to negativity regardless of how positive you are in your daily life. The only way to overcome this is to figure out the most effective actions to take when dealing with the negative feelings. Knowing that tomorrow will be better than the present can help reduce the negative impact of your life.

Make Your Choices

The inevitable changes and difficulties are there However, they won't prevent you from reaching your goals in your life. It's all about how you approach your goals. To ensure that you are striving towards your goals setting priorities is essential.

What is your top priority in your life? You may think of making your financial security your main goal however, this won't help when it comes to dealing with the stress associated with the occurrence of changes and difficulties. According to me, you should consider your health as a top priority.

In the very first chapter, I took an overview of the health problems that are caused by stress. If you do not take the necessary measures to safeguard your health, you could be struggling with any of these issues.

What are the best ways to prioritize your health when you are in this position? One way is to socialize. Being social beings, this is a step you should not miss. It will be easier to manage stress If you have someone you can depend on when you're feeling down.

It is also necessary to take care of yourself. This action is essential for dealing with both negative and positive changes. This is the way to promote confidence in yourself and self-confidence. These two aspects can assist you in learning how to cope with the changes.

Do not dwell on Social Media

When individuals face challenges or difficulties within their life, it's normal to be found using social media to seek out for comfort or guidance. This is the method to take when the difficulties are related to the loss of the job they have or the loss of loved ones. You can also compare their lives with those of their friends via social media.

In navigating through challenges and change, you need to be cautious when you use social media. Although it might seem like it's a good idea to post posts via social media sites, you have to keep in mind that you aren't able to reverse anything you publish. Even if you remove the post afterward there's a great possibility that someone took the photo.

Also, you must be aware when comparing your own life to the lives of your peers using social networks. The posts they make don't give the full image of what's happening inside their world. They are simply trying to look attractive to the world.

Nobody will post an account of the difficulties they experience behind the scenes. If you're looking for a way to overcome your problems and reduce stress, social media isn't a good location to do it.

Participate in a support Group

Your life is an athletic race. To complete this race you require the support of other people at some moment or the other. The instances when you require the assistance of others for instance, when you face difficulties and changes.

Relying on your group of friends in these situations is not an indication of weakening. It's merely an acknowledgement of your ability to realize how far you are able to go by yourself. Your support group is comprised of family members, friends and others you are able to trust.

These are the people who are happy to be at your side throughout your difficult moments. They will help you take care of your children to lessen the burden on your shoulders. You can also count on your friends and neighbors to help.

If your problems become too much you may be tempted to commit suicide. Spending time with your family and your friends can help get over these fears.

Don't fall into Denial

The majority of stress caused by changes is usually the result of trying to avoid confronting the changes. When you are denial-driven it is a great tool to delay the changes. This can make things more difficult than they need to be.

It is more difficult to suffer in the event that you deny what is taking place in your life. It's easy to imagine things to go differently. But, you need to realize that the adjustments in your life are something you'll never be able to influence.

Chapter 16: Control Your Environment

Control Of Your Environment

If you're feeling stressed the most effective thing you can do is to try to keep the control over your environment. If you aren't in control of your surroundings things can become very messy quickly. There are plenty of options to assist in calming a stressful situation. Below is a list actions you can take to manage or alter an unpleasant situation.

Tell us about your feelings. It's difficult for people around you to comprehend the feelings you're feeling if you do not share your feelings. And if they don't know what's wrong and how they can help in resolving it?

Be open to compromise. There may be a reason that it isn't exactly how you would like it to be but there must be a middle option acceptable. A majority of people will accept compromises if given the opportunity.

Manage your time. If you are stressed due to time management issues then you must master managing your time better. This is a problem which is entirely your responsibility to resolve.

Learn to accept the things aren't yours to change and then move towards the next. Be aware of the things you can alter, and then alter them.

You can forgive easily. One of the most valuable gifts you can do for yourself is the ability of forgiving others. It will help you free yourself from guilt and regret.

Always look for the positive side of any situation, even if you think there's no one. People who always find the positive in every situation are usually much happier.

You can reduce the intensity and intensity level of your feelings. If you're emotionally all in the air others will be as well. It only serves to make the situation worse. If you can manage your emotions or at least decrease them, you can help others to do the same.

Be organized. If you're organized, it will decrease stress. There's less to fret and worry about. There is no need to worry about what's happening or how you can accomplish your tasks if everything is well-organized.

Accept yourself and other people. Everyone has flaws, nobody is flawless. Accepting that can aid in understanding you and others better.

Don't overstretch yourself. There's only a limit to how many things you can manage simultaneously. Be patient, and others will get it.

Although this is merely one of the ways you can take control of your surroundings It is a good starting point. Being in control can lessen your stress. This will also help in reducing the pressure of those who are around you. When you're in control, everyone will feel more secure and the situation will be less difficult to manage.

Chapter 17: De-Stress Your Soul And Mind

Control Your Thoughts

The surrender of control

Management of stress can be a complicated phenomenon. It is essential to control something in order to regulate it, like testing your shower to determine the quantity of water hot. You turn on the water and adjust the cold and hot mixture of water to adjust the temperature. If the temperature isn't right you go through the door to shower, and begin lathering. Unfortunately, depending on your preference there is no "warm" as well as "cold" water pressure taps. It is not possible to simply turn off positive emotions and thoughts at the same time shutting off unpleasant and uncomfortable emotions.

Manage means to recognize that the various factors in any given situation are not managed and controlled. When you manage something, it is impossible to control or manage all the elements that are involved. You suffer from uncontrollableness and you continue to move towards your goal.

Although your mind is extremely helpful in coping with stressors from the outside but it could also cause stress when dealing with internal stressors. It is important to note that the brain is a continuous machine for thinking and experiencing. It is the way he is thinking and feeling. It's never off, and all the processes of it can't be managed or stopped. The effort to stop thoughts and emotions is similar to trying to stop the disappearing train. The best thing to do is to slow down the pace and pay attention to just a couple of words.

The research shows that it's getting harder to stop, control, or get rid of troubling thoughts, your own script visual images, and uncomfortable emotions. When you are focusing your entire attention and attempting to control unsettling thoughts or feelings this increases your power of mind.

You could even illustrate this with an incredibly enjoyable picture not as stressful as a vibrant white, red, or blue ball from the beach. Imagine how you feel when you throw the ball upwards and then caught by the ball as it flies back towards you. Take a deep breath and consider the glowing beach ball you toss around and down with great precision. Imagine it for a couple of seconds. You can stop thinking about it right now. I'd like you to try hard to not think about that beach ball that is bright red, blue, and white. You have to forget about that beach ball really difficult. Keep reading and then stop thinking of the ball. Do you notice what happens when you attempt to manage your beach ball? Are they gone, or have they gotten more intense? Most of the time they didn't make them disappear when you tried to manage your thoughts.

The most crucial aspect of regaining your stress is learning how to divert your attention on less-than-sad thoughts, private text messages and images of mental trauma emotional states, and behaviors that are consistent with your beliefs. This is about being better prepared to engage in positive actions and creating better environment. Control and willingness are two opposites and the more threatening thoughts and negative emotions you attempt to manage, the less likely to act. The more comfortable to tolerate unpleasant thoughts and emotions and feelings, the less to manage them so that they behave.

Control and the capacity to make decisions based on values are the most important components of reconsidering your strategy to protect yourself from stress that is accompanied by suffering and pain. It is common to get stuck and remain in a rut when you are unable to act since you have to manage all the variables in stressful situations.

How to deal with pain

It is a difficult subject to tackle and we have strong internal mechanisms that can deal with it. There are two kinds of pain you have to be aware. The one is acute pain that is not cured by awareness. It is the kind of discomfort that comes from an injury to your body or a issue that has arisen within your life. This kind of pain is a medical issue and not an emotional one.

The second type that is chronic. The cause of chronic pain might be physical, however there is an mental and emotional component that mindfulness can deal with. While removing pain can be a challenge to reduce the burden that you bear as a result of it is definitely possible. Research suggests that mindfulness and meditation methods can assist in dealing with chronic pain (Penman 2019).

While meditation is extremely efficient, applying the entire system that is based on mindfulness problem is the best strategy. How can you achieve this? First, is to first look into the cause of pain.

Step One

The typical reaction when we feel pain is to squeeze our muscles in the area which causes pain, and hope that it will go away. Our reaction is both physical and emotional element to it In the midst of pain, it's difficult to differentiate the two. Mindfulness can help you accomplish this.

Why is it crucial to distinguish the two components that trigger your reactions? For one your reactions to the pain usually cause it to be more severe than it actually is. Consider the child who slips and falls in the belief that nobody is watching. Most of the time children will clean their feet and continue running. But, if the child realizes that their parents watching and she observes their faces of fear when they run towards her, she'll undoubtedly begin crying.

In this instance the negative emotions of the parents cause an infant to assume that that his suffering is more severe than it really is. A lot of the suffering is pure emotional exaggeration. The same thing happens for us adults even if we do not shed tears. In the midst of this, we are prone to react physically to hurt in inappropriate ways .

Although clenching muscles around the pain point is a normal response but you'll notice when doing the body scan exercise that the intensity of this tension goes beyond the area affected. The clenching of muscles to this degree sends a stress signal to your brain, which consequently does what it has to.

Stress is the body's way to deal with threats that are mortal. If your brain senses the threat of death it redirects circulation of blood towards your limbs. It prioritizing certain bodily functions, for example, physical movement and breathing, to allow rapid flight, and deprioritizes other ones like digestion. This causes a huge pressure on the body. Adrenaline gets released to give you an extra boost and gives you a temporary immunity to pain.

The situation can't be sustained for long as it places an enormous burden on your internal organs and systems. If you're spending excessively in these circumstances the brain will shut down and require rest. The long-term exposure to stress can trigger stress-related disorders such as PTSD and the like. Although the strain you feel might not be to the same magnitude as an actual threat the mere presence of it puts an immense strain on your body.

By being in a state of relaxation it is possible to release the stressful interpretation of the events the brain is processing. Another method recommended by mindfulness is to feel the pain and observe the way it flows and ebbs.

Step Two

Should you be suffering whenever you feel discomfort? You should think about this problem a little longer before coming up with the answer. Pain or suffering is two distinct things. The stimulus is what causes the pain. is. It is your response to the discomfort. With this in mind, ask yourself: is it really necessary to endure in discomfort?

The answer is simple: that it's not. In actuality, however it's hard to live in this manner. We're accustomed to mixing our pain with our feelings of pain, so that they form one cohesive reaction. Mindfulness will help you discern these two. The first thing to consider is whether you are experiencing any barriers to letting your emotions flow.

We're taught many ways to express our emotions. These range from having a rational outlook toward things to completely disproving the authenticity of our feelings. The most common advice is to be able to accept emotions and let them flow. Unfortunately, this is not enough.

Acknowledgement needs to be coupled with acceptance in order for it to be effective. Mere acknowledgement simply means acknowledging the existence of emotions, but does not mean that you are engaging with them. The same way, letting your emotions flow gives them time to breathe but to not be in contact with them any more.

It is important to be able to allow your emotions to go through you. The most important thing to do is to be aware of your decision in responding to your emotions. Through observing and trying to be calm and calmness, you can improve your ability to handle discomfort and separate emotions from the stimuli. Thus, you'll be able to feel the pain, but should not exacerbate your pain by reacting in a way that is inappropriate to it.

Step Three

3. The most crucial step is to establish your goals to live your life now in the present. Only

focus on what's being revealed to you now Don't think about what it will mean in the future. If you're suffering from suffering right now take care of it right now. If it comes up in the future take care of it immediately.

In this instance, suppose you fall on something very badly, you feel the pain as well as feel negative emotions rising up within you. It is painful, and your feelings are legitimate. Do not try to keep them in a bottle. Try to distinguish the physical sensation from your emotional reaction however, if you're unable to accomplish this, don't be worried about it.

It's possible to be concerned in case you're bleeding. You should check to determine whether you're bleeding. Are you worried that you're bleeding the thought that you'll have to visit the hospital to get examined, and then thinking about how much it's going to cost and how much time you'll have to put into doing this will only add to your pain.

It is also a way to travel in the past to see what could take place. Mindfulness demands that you remain in the present moment and observe what happens. Be aware of your feelings and let your emotions run free. When you're done, get back to the task you started and get back to work. When you are feeling pain be aware of it and begin to learn to appreciate it. This is aspect of life in the end and you can't enjoy life without suffering. Accept it and let it be a part of your life.

Tips to decrease negative thoughts

Do not think too much.

There's nothing more maniacal and unattractive than thinking too much. If you are constantly thinking your thoughts, your brain isn't in its most optimal state. Your motivations may differ in the course of your day it is possible to not know what your priorities are. This is common with the kind of attitude.

One of the best ways to not to get caught up in thoughts is to set aside time for you to be meditative. A mere 20 minutes of meditation each day can help you break down the negative thoughts that plague you and allow you to concentrate on what is important. Try it for several weeks and observe the changes in your patterns of over-thinking.

Watch out for chances to win, but not a problem

Writers are extremely sensitive team. We are prone to be very negative, and we also focus on the problems and are enslaved by them.

This can make us susceptible to seeing and interpreting everything. Every single thing that happens to us each day including rejections, to not being able to finish our word count We translate all of these things into negative consequences.

When we shift our mindset from negative to positive ones, and look at every challenge as an opportunity for learning and improvement in our performance, our cognitive abilities improve and we show an opportunity to be seen as to be happier and productive. There are courses that are embedded in every single one of these topics. We all wish to do is take advantage of in a way that allows us to determine the course they've taken.

Refrain from negative thoughts with

Sometimes, we're our very self-defence. We are able to focus on our negative thoughts through the actions we're taking. This can lead to patterns of negative thinking which could last for a considerable time in the absence of being attentive. It is therefore important for authors to avoid destructive thoughts from getting in their ways. Rememberthat you're new to the world trying to manage a difficult environment. It's possible but it's quite difficult initially.

If you follow this advice by following this advice, you'll surely be taking good steps to avoid negative thoughts and attitudes. This can boost your creativity and overall productivity. Also, this could be a win-win situation for the majority of writers and other outside.

Control your emotions

How to identify emotions

The way you react to emotions is how you react to an event. It's not an easy job to do as it takes patience and time. Different people experience different emotions. You must take your time you to recognize the appropriate emotion.

Then, why do you be able to identify emotions at all? They are divided into three parts that are the subjective, physical, and expressive components. The subjective component is the way you feel emotion while the physiological component relates to how your body responds to emotion, and the expressive component is about how you react to emotion.

These elements play an important part in the way you react to emotions.

The role that emotions are playing in our lives

They encourage us to act

The way you feel affects how you react to situations. For instance, if you have to take an examination, you'll be worried about how you'll perform and how the exam can affect the result you receive. Due to the reactions you could be pressured to improve your studying. The emotions allow you to perform a task and improve the results.

They also let us choose the actions we should undertake; generally these actions are aimed to help us feel more positive emotions and lessen the chance of experiencing negative emotions.

The emotions we feel help us to survive

It is through emotions that allow us to stay safe as well as to stay alive and reproduce. When we feel upset, the instinct is usually to address the issue. If we're afraid of being confronted, we're likely to flee.

The role of emotions is encouraging us to take action fast, which can boost the odds of success and longevity.

They assist us in making decisions

The emotions of our lives can influence the decisions we take. For example, when we are angry and want to find an opportunity to improve the situation. Even in the event of circumstances that require us to choose solely on the basis of logic and reason but we still operate on emotions.

Emotions help us communicate

When we speak to others, it is essential that we provide them with clues to help them comprehend our message better. These clues are based on emotions, which are then displayed through our body language. It could be in the appearance of facial expressions which are linked to specific emotions we feel.

In certain instances it may require us to express our feelings in a direct manner. For example, if we inform someone that we feel unhappy, happy or scared, we have eaten, providing them with crucial information could be used to act.

They help us understand the thoughts of others.

In the same way that we give people an impression of what we are feeling by displaying our emotions and the feelings of other people can also provide us with an insight into what others are thinking or planning to do.

If we can recognize and understand emotions, we will can react to their feelings in the right way. If we are educated about emotions, we can react in the correct manner towards them, which results in better interactions with others.

Chapter 18: Continue Activities With Positive

A lot of people are prone to avoid their normal activities when they're overwhelmed, anxious, or depressed. They are afraid to take on too much stimulation and tend to prefer being alone. A tendency to stay away from social activities can be harmful to the condition, particularly those suffering from depression. Sometimes , it is difficult to get back on track and get out to a social gathering or even a lunch with your friend However, the health benefits you reap after you've made the decision are typically immediate.

In addition to the relief from stress Socializing is also proven to boost your immune system and help fight the flu and cold, and could even aid in living longer. Socializing, particularly in seniors, keeps their brains stimulated and lowers the chance to develop dementia. In the case of stress, participating in activities that involve social interaction boosts your mood and assists in distracting you from the stressors, even at least for a brief period of time. Spend time with your friends and clear your thoughts off of the things that stress you out. It's easy to get lost in your thoughts. The longer you think about those negative feelings, the larger they get. One caviot is there but. People you surround yourself with must be positive friendly people. Being around people who just want to complain about their issues and snark about their fellow members and have nothing to provide other than negativity is not going to reduce stress levels. Sometimes, it's necessary to leave your circle of acquaintances to find some relief. Here are some ideas to try:

Participate in an exercise class: A bonding session with a new person during your workout class is a fantastic opportunity to break the cold. You're both here to make a difference and enhance your health. Try to say hello or introduce yourself a person within the group. They may be seeking someone new to connect with. Even if you never speak to someone you've never met attending a class could provide you with the feeling of being part of a community that you won't experience from making a video exercise at home, or even taking an outing on your own. The entire class is doing exactly the same thing, and they are doing it voluntarily. As a result, you share something, which can aid in the formation of new friendships.

If you are socially better you should consider joining a sports team if there is enough time. Team sports like softball or volleyball keeps your mind and body engaged and constantly communicating with your team. You'll celebrate victories together while you train together and create new friendships.

Volunteer: Whether that's in your community soup kitchen, or helping with the planning of the event of your choice, getting involved can bring you joy since you're helping others. You'll likely being able to share your time with other like-minded people who are eager to help too.

Being active in your community can bring you in contact with someone who you've not yet met. Making friends in your community will provide you with the opportunity to talk to someone when you're having trouble. It is also a chance to learn new techniques that will improve confidence in yourself and your mood. Every aspect of it suggests that stress relief is in the air.

If you're unsure of where to start look on bulletin boards in the community and the local newspaper for notices of events coming up and requests for volunteers. You could be involved in coordinating your town's parade repairing something, or collecting donations for families in need. Choose a cause that appeals to you and the task doesn't feel like work. Remember that the main ingredient to stress relief is to do something that you enjoy to increase your endorphins. It should not make you feel more stressed. As we mentioned before, the over-extension of yourself can be an issue that causes stress. Be sure that the volunteer project you select to take part in is a good fit within your daily schedule and doesn't require more commitment than you are willing to give. A single volunteer opportunity is the ideal way to start. For example, raking leaves on the town green is likely to take just a few hours, with no commitment. This gives you the chance to go out and enjoy yourself without making a long-term commitment.

Networking events: The majority of people view networking events as a means to connect with their colleagues or find the acquaintance of new clients for their company. It might not be an effective way to ease stress when your primary concern is at work. Even though most events are geared towards work-related topics, there is a chance to connect with individuals in different ways.

For starters, getting to know your colleagues or those working in the same field as you will have benefits. If you decide to go to one of these events you should only talk about your work and spend a period of time trying to know them in a way that is personal. The people who you meet don't want to work for long hours as well. Additionally, getting to get to know someone may bring you new customers and make you an approachable, likable human being. If the primary cause of stress is anxiety over social situations or networking, then carrying on conversations with strangers can cause your blood pressure to increase. The goal is to ease stress, keep in mind that often facing the issue face-to-face is the only method to address the issue and reduce stress. Many people find that talking isn't a natural thing. It requires the ability to think and focus to be able to do it. Consider networking as a skill for the job (because it truly is). You didn't learn to operate a computer at work in a day but eventually you learned. The more you work at communicating with other people, the better you'll become and less stress-inducing it will be.

If your work activities don't sound appealing, consider your most loved pastime. For example, let's say you love knitting or other crafts. Look for craft fairs or a local knitting groups. Connecting with people who share similar interests is a fantastic method to get conversations going, and boost your endorphins. Learning new knowledge from new acquaintances can help boost your self-confidence as well. You may even make some new friends. Play with your pet If social interaction with humans holds no appeal for you, especially if a significant part of your anxiety comes from social anxiety then starting with a pet can be a great way to way to transition. Engaging with a cat or dog is more relaxing than having an exchange with a human. Pets are just as happy to play, be pet and cuddle. Even when they do get agitated and talk to each other, they do not interrupt and help relieve anxiety.

If you own already got a pet, make sure you spend quality time together. Go for a long stroll, play in the backyard or simply take the time to appreciate and acknowledge the fact that they're there. Keep in mind that your dog is always eager to meet you once you return back home, regardless of whether you've missed a crucial meeting at work or did not. They aren't concerned about anything, except for you. Remember this frequently when you work to boost your spirits. Consider how they sway around, wave their tails, and kiss your face to greet you when you enter the building. It gives you something to anticipate. Cats are wonderful too however their affection isn't as enthusiastic. They might just rub against your leg or snuggle close to you on the sofa However, the affection is exactly the same. Numerous studies have proven that pet owners suffer less anxiety, less blood pressure, and a lower chance of developing depression.

Going with your dog to the park or taking walks can also draw others who love dogs. As it is crucial for your dog to interact with other dogs, so too you must be socializing with their owners as well. Conversations that are simple can result in play dates, laughter and even the possibility of making a new friend. If you do not have pets, you could be thinking about buying one, but be aware that having a pet requires an investment of time and money. Don't adopt a pet if you do not have the time for the animal, as it is likely to suffer. Instead, consider volunteering at the local shelter for animals. You can interact with and walk dogs, or cuddle with kittens and cats. Although you're not committed to them in the long run but you can brighten their day and yours, by spending some quality time together.

Chapter 19: Reaching Out

It can be difficult to share with others your feelings, however, it is an act of courage and not asking for assistance or help could be counterproductive. In the workplace, if your bosses don't know that you're stressed out, they can't do anything to assist you or ease the stress the cause of your anxiety. They are only able to assist when they know.

If the level of stress and emotional turmoil is such that you're unable speak to family, friends or colleagues at work, then perhaps it's time to see your doctor for advice and assistance.

Laughter

A good laugh makes every day a more enjoyable one for you to be. But, not many people plan to enjoy laughter. We'd rather spend the evening in the evening, watching politically-oriented programs that fill our minds with bad news and conflict instead of making an effort to read, listen to or see something entertaining.

My wife and I during the past year, have decided to go out and enjoy ourselves more and, in the process, have witnessed some amazing stand-up comedy. It led me to doing stand-up comedy for myself during an open mic night ...... in the event that you could describe what I did as comedy!

Laughter is a high-speed broadband connection to your body's happiness-inducing chemical mix. Endorphins are a rush along with the release and release of the hormone oxytocin triggered by laughter could make every stressor disappear into distance while you laugh away your troubles even if the relief lasts only a few minutes.

Have fun! .... Enjoy a laugh !

Music

For most individuals, it's true that music has the potential to be a great motivational tool, however most of us don't make use of music beyond leisure time. At school, I've seen increasing numbers of schools removing alarms and bells and substituting them with music that slowly becomes louder (or soft) that prepares the brain for breaks or lessons, and gives everyone , including teachers time to prepare to start or finish of the break-time or class instead of the silence which is broken by the snarling bell or alarm. What about replacing the alarm clock you use to wake up with a mood alarm that , 5 minutes prior to your wake up time, it begins to play relaxing or upbeat classical music as the gradually brighter light appears? A nighttime time with these clocks can be equally relaxing when the light gradually fades away to a soft piece of music that eases your mind and helps you sleep.

If you're an instrument player then why not play every day even if just for just ten minutes. A majority of people discover that when they're focused on their instrument, it is nearly impossible to be distracted by other issues in an end of the head because your mind is focused on the work of making music. It is also a fantastic method of changing the negative "state" by creating oxygen and exercising the facial muscles (regardless of how great an artist is ... or aren't). There's nothing more enjoyable than singing a tune with a high voice that makes you feel content. What number of times do you stopped at the traffic light to look at the vehicle in front of you and observe people who are putting in their best when they belt out their favorite song that's been playing from the radio? Do you ask yourself: ...... Do they appear at ease or stressed? Do you dare? .... I dare you! (but take care to watch the road, eh?).

Music can be a great way to relieve stress. So whether you're a professional performer or not which I'm not (I was designed to be comfortable, not fast) So why not turn on some tunes and dance as if no one is watching you. Maybe you could attend dance classes and enjoy an evening out with your friends or your partner?

In any case music can be a great way to unwind from the pressures of daily life.

Relaxation for the eyes with closed-eyes

It's okay. We've examined the factors, causes of stress, the symptoms, and the consequences of stress. We've also examined numerous strategies for preventing stress which you can use to change your life. The exercise of closing your eyes is one of the most important ways you can lessen your stress.

As explained in the beginning chapter, you should first try recording yourself (if feasible) talking the process in such a way that when you're ready to relax, you will listen to "your personal voice" encouraging you to take a break. While doing this exercise, remember be sure not to operate machines or drive. If you are suffering from epilepsy, make sure you remain alert during the exercise.

The closed-eye exercise is an autogenic procedure that allows you to relax from head to the toe. It is a good idea to think about your muscles relaxed all the way from top to bottom, and after the exercise you will be energized yourself and feel great when you return. What I'd like you to do is to lie down on the floor or on the bed or sit in a comfy spot. Your arms and legs must be separated and your limbs should not touch one another, by that I mean that your arms should be a little bit away from your body, and your legs should be separated. If you're in an office chair take a seat in a straight-backed chair with your back lying flat against the rear of the chair with your feet set firmly on the floor. Your arms should be placed in your laps or across your hips which ever is more comfortable for you. Whether you're lying down or sitting in a chair, be aware that you've got your hands twisted into fists, toes , or teeth clenched. If they are, let them relax. Take note of whether you've got particular tight clothes around your wrist, waist or neck, and if you do you can loosen them. Be aware of whether you are grinding or clenching your teeth or grinding your teeth, in which case let your jaw let itself relax. If you have to be awake at a specific time, in case you are prone to falling asleep, you should set alarms on your phone or computer or on a timer close by , so that if want to, you'll be awakened at the exact time you're required to. If you have to open your eyes due to any reason, you'll be able to take a step back and be alert and alert and be remain in complete and safe control at any point.

Be sure to .... Go through the book first, and then take notes of the process before applying for yourself, the procedure to relax. The next step is more lengthy than the first.

Also... In case you have epilepsy, make sure you be sure to keep your eyes open (of of course, you can blink) If your condition is more than mild or if you suffer from "any" medical issue which might make you unfit for the method I strongly recommend that you consult with your doctor prior to performing any closed-eye relaxation procedure. This could include but isn't limited to heart issues blood pressure issues and psychological or emotional issues as well as chest or lung health concerns, seizures or fits of any kind. For all other people the result is much more favorable by closing your eyes while listening to the audio that I'm soliciting to record.

Record of the Press:

Be conscious about your breath. Do you feel it is very shallow from the chest's high point or do you breathe very deep from the stomach pit?

Take note that you breathe.

I'd like you to be in control of your breathing, and to be more conscious the quality of your air.

Be aware of what you observe, as you begin to control your breathing. You begin to take deep, long breaths. With each breath, hold your breath for just a few seconds before exhaling and letting loose the tension in the muscles ...... and let them relax.

Every time you breathe out you can relax immer more at ease.

Each breath you take let yourself ease into a deeper relaxation, releasing any tension that remains especially around your neck and shoulder areas.

Keep in mind that at any moment or at any time you are able to take a step forward and remain aware, awake, and responsive to any circumstance that requires you to act accordingly.

However, for the moment, continue taking a few deep breaths, allowing yourself to rest even more and allow your eyes to slowly close, if you want to as you unwind in silence.

In a second we'll be counting from five to one. Take deep breaths and continue to take long, deep breaths for each number we take in, but allow yourself to take a break and relax even more.

Let yourself float and sink deeper into a secure, comfortable state of bliss.

Five:

Imagine the muscles at both sides of your head and forehead relax, let go of tension as you slowly sink deeper and more deeply into a state of relaxation.

Four:

Relax the muscles that surround your cheek bones, the upper back of your head, neck. Feel your chin relaxed and relax.

Every breath you take exhale, releasing tension. You will feel all facial muscles relax even more.

As you continue to sink, allow yourself the freedom to relax while your shoulders' muscles ease.

Three:

Continue to relax every breath you take and the upper chest area, the back, and then down to your stomach , towards your waistline along your sides, and back. .... Every time you breathe out, you'll feel more at ease.

Two:

Continue to go downwards... then downwards, drifting, floating to a area of complete relaxation relaxing the tension of your waist muscles along with your bottom and legs.

One;

Deeper breaths then hold for 3 minutes. When you exhale, allow the sensation of relaxation be felt from your head to your thighs, removing any tension and easing you further.

Next, breathe through your thighs, circling your knees, and then your calf muscles as well as your shins.

After your next breath, to your ankles, float further down, still relaxing in a drift and allowing yourself to ease tension in your muscles.

You are welcome to take an hour or so to relax and enjoy your secure peaceful, tranquil state.

(allow the silence to last for about 20-30 secs or so)

Now, focus upon your breathing. deepen your breaths and out. With each breath, allow you to feel more alert.

In the next moment, we'll count from one to five. At every count, take a deep and long breath that allows more oxygen to enter your body. You will hold it for two seconds while allowing yourself to feel bit more awake and awake and alert.

One,

Take a long , deep breath, take it in for 2 seconds. Then allow yourself to be conscious of the surroundings.

Two,

Take a long, deep breath and hold it for a few seconds, and then begin to experience a stretching, maybe tighten the muscles a more in your arms. Then let them relax again.

Three,

Take a long, deep breath.

You could start to wiggle your toes as well as moving your mouth. those facial muscles .... simply inject some energy into them. You will also become more aware of your surroundings , including being aware of the seat or floor below you. You will become more alert, lively and alert.

Four,

Inhale deeply, take a long breath, then gradually open your eyes on the count of five . after a few breaths, let you to become more aware, alert and energetic.

Move your limbs around and maybe do a stretch, and then be ready for five to be able to see and at your own pace when it's appropriate for you to do this get up and do some stretch. Return fully energized alert and alert.

Five,

take a deep breath, smile, and smile at yourself take a deep breath, and at your own pace, when it's safe and comfortable to do this take a few minutes to stretch or stroll around, and then return to your routine feeling rejuvenated.

Press STOP:

Conclusion

The management of stress is definitely under your control. There are instances that you feel overwhelmed. If you decide to examine what's your issue in an objective manner, the odds of finding solutions that work for your concerns are good. In order to find solutions that work your mind and body must be at ease and free of anxiety and stress. A relaxed mind and body can make a difference.

Recognizing, accepting and acknowledging the existence in stress are the initial step to take to control it. Once you have passed this initial phase there are numerous ways to deal with anxiety and stress. Find methods that work for your requirements and that fit with your daily routine.

Explore the methods in this book one at a and then select a few or more that work best for you and your requirements. It is essential to apply relaxation and stress management techniques until they become a habit that is ingrained in your mind. This is crucial because the demands of modern society and the expectations from you will continue to get more demanding.

www.ingramcontent.com/pod-product-compliance
Lightning Source LLC
Chambersburg PA
CBHW071124130526
44590CB00056B/1904